Am I Ready?

Teen Girls Write About Sex

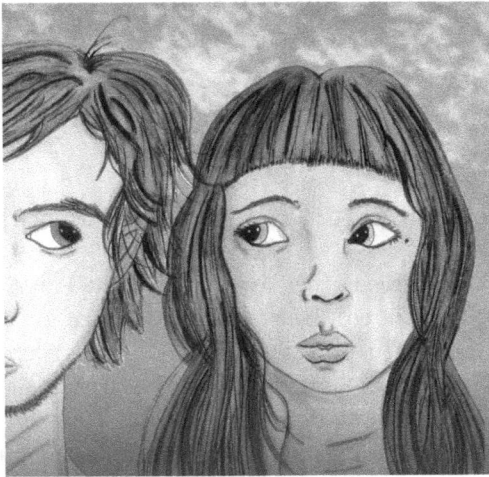

By Youth Communication

Edited by Virginia Vitzthum

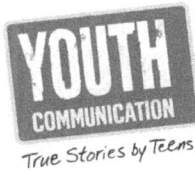

YOUTH COMMUNICATION

True Stories by Teens

Am I Ready?

EXECUTIVE EDITORS
Keith Hefner and Laura Longhine

CONTRIBUTING EDITORS
Andrea Estepa, Nora McCarthy, Tamar Rothenberg,
Clarence Haynes, Hope Vanderberg, Rachel Blustain,
Al Desetta, Philip Kay, and Katia Hetter

LAYOUT & DESIGN
Efrain Reyes, Jr. and Jeff Faerber

PRODUCTION
Stephanie Liu

COVER ART
Rosangel Dagnesses

For reprint information, please contact Youth Communication.

ISBN 978-1-935552-30-7

Second, Expanded Edition

Printed in the United States of America

Youth Communication ®
New York, New York
www.youthcomm.org

Catalog Item #YD21-1

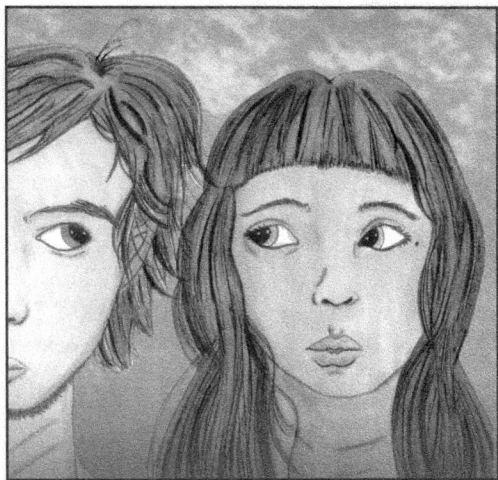

Table of Contents

Womanhood Can Wait

Nicole Hawkins..13

*Most girls are in a hurry to grow up, but Nicole wants
to take it slow.*

I Stopped Giving in to Him

Anonymous..20

*After years of experiencing sex as a tedious duty, the
writer realizes she has the right to say no.*

When It Comes to Dating, Older Isn't Better

Shaniece McKenzie...27

*Shaniece explores the issue of teen girls having sex
with older guys, and concludes that these relationships
can be risky for girls.*

Communication Is More Important Than Sex

Anonymous..31

*The writer shares her concerns about sex with her
boyfriend, and he agrees to wait until she's ready.
When they do decide to have sex, it feels special.*

Virgin Under Pressure

Anonymous..36

*The writer feels pressured to have sex by her boyfriend,
and almost gives in before she realizes she's not ready.*

The Morning After

Anonymous 44

Caught up in the heat of the moment, the writer has unprotected sex one night. The next morning she's terrified she may be pregnant.

Looking for Love

Fetima P. 50

Devastated after her father leaves the family, Fetima fills her emptiness by losing her virginity at 13 and having promiscuous sex. As she gets older, she reflects on her behavior and gains control of her sexuality.

I Need a Girl

Destiny 56

Destiny is 13 when she realizes she's attracted to women, but isn't sure she's gay until she meets Keesha.

All Men Are Dawgs

Wunika Hicks 60

Wunika reflects on the double standard that condemns women who play the field but not men.

I Was Scared but I Wanted Experience

Anonymous 64

Eager to get "experience," the writer rushes into sex with a boy she hardly knows.

Can We Talk About Sex With Our Parents?

Anonymous 72

> The writer interviews other teens about how they talk
> to their parents about sex — and discovers that most
> aren't talking about it at all.

Dirty Dancing

Janill Briones 77

> Janill is appalled by the openly sexual "dancing" that
> goes on at her school dance.

It Takes Love to Make Love

Anonymous 81

> The writer, 15, is pressured into having sex and feels
> disillusioned by the experience. Later she realizes sex
> can be physically and emotionally satisfying with the
> right person.

Single, Happy, and Free

Irma Johnson 89

> Irma finds that many teens are perfectly happy not
> dating and don't feel they're missing anything.

The Right Choice—for Now

Anonymous 92

> The writer, 17, becomes pregnant in her sophomore
> year of high school and struggles to decide what to do.

Scare Tactics

Anonymous...97
   The writer has mixed feelings about abortion, but she
   believes all women should be able to make their own
   decision without intimidation.

I Paid the Price for Unprotected Sex—Twice

Anonymous...102
   After contracting chlamydia for the second time, the
   writer resolves to start protecting herself.

Sexually Transmitted Diseases:
Protect Yourself and Your Partner 106

FICTION SPECIAL: Someone to Love Me

Anne Schraff..109

Using the Book

Teens: How to Get More Out of This Book........................118

How to Use This Book in Staff Training 119

Teachers & Staff: How to Use This Book in Groups 120

Credits.. 122

About Youth Communication 123

About the Editors.. 126

More Helpful Books from Youth Communication 128

Introduction

Sex may be the most confusing thing in a girl's life. Whether to have it and, if so, who to have it with are huge decisions. And those decisions are complicated by so many things: trust in your partner, protecting yourself from pregnancy and STDs/STIs, worries about your reputation, listening to your own body and heart to know what you really want. The writers in this book cover this strange, overwhelming world with great honesty, self-awareness, and perception.

For some of the writers, sex simply does not live up to the hype. As the anonymous writer of "I Stopped Giving in to Him," puts it, "Most of my experiences with sex have had very little to do with love and care." She is one of several writers who report back lessons learned the hard way. After she tells the boy who impregnated her that she had an abortion, "'Oh' is all he said to me, like I was just one more girl that he had knocked up."

This writer concludes, as many of the girls in this book do, that she needs to take more control over her sexuality and relationships. "I know, now, that if I don't want to have sex, then I don't have to. I will only truly enjoy sex if I do it when I'm ready. If my man can't handle that and he wants to leave then it wasn't meant to be between us, and I still have time to find the right guy for me."

Other writers come to the same conclusion without having sex. The anonymous writer of "Virgin Under Pressure" admits she likes boys pushing her for sex because it makes her feel desirable. But after several scary encounters where she feels disrespected, she concludes, "I think my best option is not to have sex while I'm still in high school. I do want to have sex someday, but I want to do it with someone who respects me and who will be there for me for a long time."

Another difficult aspect of sex is the collision of honesty and privacy. Even adults tend to be private about their sex lives, and teens especially may feel forced to lie. In "Can We Talk About Sex With Our Parents?" the author interviews other teens and finds that many of them share her fear of bringing up the subject with a parent.

Some writers in this book face some of sex's more concrete dangers: unwanted pregnancy and sexually transmitted diseases. The anonymous writer of "Scare Tactics" describes feeling pressured and confused by what she heard in an anti-abortion clinic. Another anonymous writer tells about getting chlamydia, and the book's final piece gives an overview of STDs—how they're transmitted, how to protect against them, and how to treat them.

The sex news isn't all grim, though. The anonymous writer of "Sex With the Wrong Guy" does find the right guy and gets closer to him through sex. She only arrives there, though, after she's learned to place her own wishes above anyone else's and held out for a boy who respects and likes her. In "When It Comes to Dating, Older Isn't Better," Shaniece McKenzie leaves readers with simple advice that applies both to girls who are waiting and to those who aren't: "Keep it real with yourself, and think about what's right for you."

In the following stories, names and/or identifying details have been changed: *I Stopped Giving in to Him, Communication Is More Important than Sex, Virgin Under Pressure, The Morning After, I Need a Girl, I Was Scared but I Wanted Experience, Can We Talk About Sex With Our Parents?* and *Sex With the Wrong Guy.*

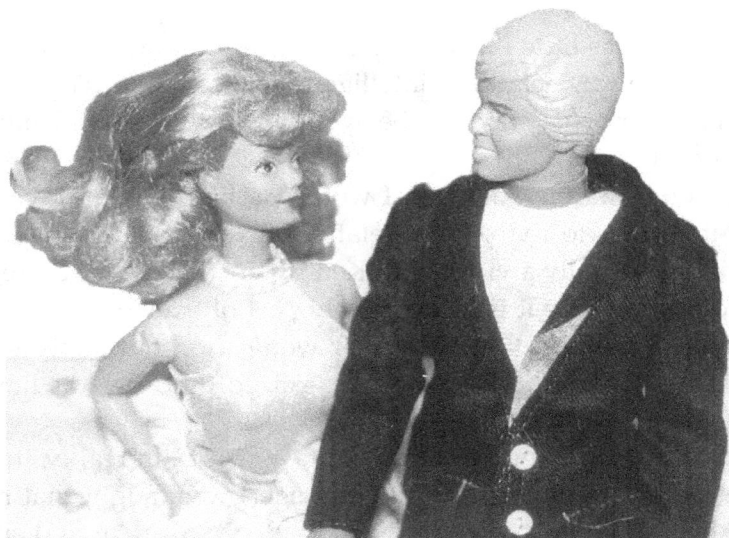

YC Art Dept.

Womanhood Can Wait

By Nicole Hawkins

Sometimes, when I'm walking down the block, I'll see a 12-year-old girl wearing revealing, sexy clothes, and I'll wonder if this little girl knows something more than I know. What inside of her makes her want to possess and flaunt such sexuality when it is too much for me to deal with? I wonder why she's in a rush to capture something that seems so much bigger than the two of us: womanhood.

I am 18 years old, but I'm not exactly sure if I'm an 18-year-old woman or an 18-year-old girl. Lots of times I feel like I'm on my way. But other times I feel clueless, like everything is still new and a mystery to me. It seems like girls are always in a hurry to grow up and become women—and part of being a woman means having boyfriends and having sex. But I'm still struggling to understand who I am, and I'm not sure I'm ready for womanhood yet.

When I was little I loved to play Barbies. Barbie was her own woman. She was beautiful, intelligent, and powerful. My Barbie was a teacher by day and a babe by night. She was sexy, feminine, and proud.

Through Barbie and Ken, I would act out making love and how it related to the perfect relationship. When they had sex, Barbie was usually a virgin and Ken wasn't. She wouldn't regret it, though, because it was the final big act of true love. Later she would feel nervous that her father would find out and disown her, but when he did find out, he realized that she was happy, and just loved and supported her.

That was love and sex in my fantasy world. In reality, things were more complicated. At a young age I was taught that boys were bad while girls were nice and made up of sugar and spice. I was told to defend myself against boys any way I knew how, including scratching their eyeballs out.

My Barbie was usually a virgin and Ken wasn't.

One day when I was 6 years old, I was sitting on the couch with my legs spread wide apart. For no apparent reason my father slapped them shut. This was my first lesson on sex: It's bad to sit with your legs open.

I was told that if I had sex before I got married, I would be disowned and put in a home. Maybe my father felt that since he waited until he was about 22 years old to have sex with my mother, I, a female, should have no problem holding out. My mother was even worse. If I had sex before marriage, I would not only be considered a disappointment, but worst of all, a SLUT!

Despite these lectures, I was still very close to my father. Besides instilling fear in me, my father built up my self-esteem and taught me to do things for myself. He would say things like, "You have to do well in school so that you can be accepted into a good college, so you can be your own woman and won't have to depend on a man," and I believed him.

He taught me to depend on myself. At the same time, he made me feel like it was OK to be a kid. Even after I started dating, my father still bought me Barbie doll stuff to add to my collection. I remember feeling happy, relieved and confused all at the same time. While I was facing the idea that sooner or later I had to grow up, here was my daddy telling me, "It's OK to be a kid for as long as you can."

When I was 8 years old, my 11-year-old sister, Tamika, started puberty. It seemed like such a dreadful thing. Yuck, the acne, PMS, cramps, awkwardness, boobs, and BOYS. It just reinforced all the things my father had told me. Growing up was not fun.

It was supposed to mean taking responsibility for yourself and your actions. Instead I watched my sister's body and emotions control her, and then I watched her get grounded for acting irresponsibly. With Barbie and Ken, love was safe and predictable. But in the real-life situations my sister was experiencing, everything seemed like a tailspin.

I watched my sister become involved with boys and get hurt—either dumped or cheated on—and it made me glad that my turn was ages away. What a joy, I thought, to be able to lie on my stomach and be comfortable because my chest was completely flat. Part of me wanted to remain a little girl always.

Still, all around me people were maturing. By junior high school, the rest of my peers seemed to be well into their third or fourth relationship. I felt like something was wrong with me, unnatural. I felt like it was my duty to act mature, so I went a little boy crazy myself.

I had already had my first kiss when my mother decided to explore the pages of my diary. She called me a slut and a harlot and threatened to put me in a home. I was terrified by her reaction but a part of me wanted to show her what rebellion really was. Then something happened that stopped me dead in my tracks.

My friend Sharnette and I used to hang out and get ourselves into these fine little messes. When we were 13, Sharnette started dating this guy Ricky. Ricky had a friend, Edgar, who wanted to get hooked up with me. Edgar was cute and four years older than me. So Sharnette and I visited the boys at Ricky's house.

Edgar and I sat on the bed and talked and played video games. Then we started to kiss. Soon Edgar began to massage my breasts. Immediately I wanted to put an end to the situation, but before I could act he was pulling the ends of my shirt out of my pants.

I began to panic. I had no idea where this was going. I stood up in a rush and proclaimed that I was leaving. A couple of months later I found out that Edgar was planning to have sex with me that evening.

After that, I became fearful of guys and all my parents' warnings raced through my head. Foolishly, I'd believed I was mature enough to handle a situation that was way over my head. I started to see guys as the unpredictable, conniving creatures my father described. I still wanted to explore my sexuality, but I didn't feel safe anymore.

By the time high school started, I was also feeling more self-conscious about my body. The summer before high school, I grew a few inches and my chest swelled up to a C cup. While lots of teenage girls like attention from the opposite sex, I didn't.

I hated when guys would stare at my chest and look to see if I had a nice ass. I wore baggy jeans and plaid shirts big enough to hide the protruding obstacles settled in my bra. I became extremely shy around everyone, especially boys. For the first couple of years of high school, I don't think I even said a full sentence.

Even though I was having a really hard time, I also did a lot of growing. Being alone so much gave me space and time to explore who I was and would ultimately become. I started to become my own leader, dancing to the beat of my drum.

When I was around 14, I began to question my father's beliefs. I'd tell my father that I didn't know if I could wait until I got married to have sex. He thought I was in a rebellious, disrespectful stage. He was partially right, but not fully. I also really wanted answers about sex. I didn't want to be told that I was too young to understand, so I turned to other sources.

I started reading a lot of fashion magazines. They were full of images of new "Barbies" for me to marvel at. On the radio I discovered "Love Phones," a call-in show about sex and relationships. I would tune in every Monday through Thursday and listen to the host talk about topics such as homosexuality, AIDS, cheating, virginity, femininity, even different sexual positions.

Finding stability in other areas of my life helped me feel comfortable about my body and my sexuality.

Over the next couple of years, I began to gain control of my life. My schoolwork improved, I became very spiritual for a while, and I felt like I was rediscovering myself. I also began to feel that the sexuality that was sprouting in me was natural and shouldn't be looked upon as evil.

Last fall, I entered an alternative school and soared academically. I even joined the school newspaper. I was really confident and proud of myself. I also had a job. By finding stability in other areas of my life, I was able to begin feeling comfortable about my body and my sexuality.

For the first time in a long time I felt comfortable enough to allow myself to be emotionally vulnerable. I was ready to take on the responsibility of relationships. Soon I developed friendships with males and I no longer felt threatened.

This past year, my senior year of high school, I have really transformed. I have been living with my best friend and her family for a year because there were just too many arguments at home, and my parents agreed it would be better. I have also been working. I'm not completely independent, but for the first time in my life I feel somewhat in control and really liberated.

When I first moved in with my friend, I still wore baggy pants and no makeup. But I noticed that after my 18th birthday, my pants began to get tighter, my shirts began to get smaller, and I began to stare into the mirror, practicing and perfecting lining my lips.

There are times these days when I'll put on a dress and suddenly I'll feel more powerful. Occasionally you'll see me walking down the street, strutting with such self-confidence you wouldn't even recognize me. Sometimes dressing feminine can do that to a person.

The other day I found myself in a store looking at lingerie. That's something I'd never thought I would be doing before the Second Coming of Christ. I am actually considering buying a matching bra and panty set even though the price is too high.

A little voice inside my head is telling me, "You'll look so sexy and cute in this outfit, you'll be irresistible." Part of me wants to be in the spotlight showing everyone just how beautiful I can be.

Still, I often question the pros and cons of exhibiting my femininity. It seems like it could make me more powerful, more me. But I also worry if it will make me more passive and more likely to rely on beauty to get by.

And sometimes I'll be sitting on the train and I'll look at the professionally dressed women and I'll wonder, "What if they're as confused about themselves and life as I am? What if they're just putting on a show to make their colleagues, families, and friends believe they are Woman?" I used to believe that after your teens, you get it all down pat. But as I approach adulthood, I don't find that to be true at all.

My current boyfriend and I started dating a week after this past Valentine's Day. With Jamil it was different from the start. Even before we started dating, we were friends. We would listen to each other and make each other laugh.

And after we began going out, it was incredible. For the first time in my life I actually trusted a guy almost 100%. That was something I never thought I would do.

Even though I love Jamil and I can pretty much see myself being with him long term, I don't want to do something I'm not ready for. I have all the time in the world to experience sex. I figure, why not wait a while and experience my virginity? I still have a lot to figure out.

I know that my first time will be very intense and will make me feel vulnerable, but I don't want to feel overwhelmed or too out of control of the situation. I want it to be satisfying.

I'm glad that I've decided to be cautious about the choices I make. I'm glad that I've waited and not rushed into sex, because I haven't found myself yet. I'm not at the place I want to be.

If you asked me right now, "What do you consider yourself to be?" I'd answer that I am a bystander, a sort of misfit, searching for my place. I'm in the midst of development. I'm like a butterfly emerging from her cocoon. I hope my metamorphosis will be a revolution.

Nicole was 18 when she wrote this story.

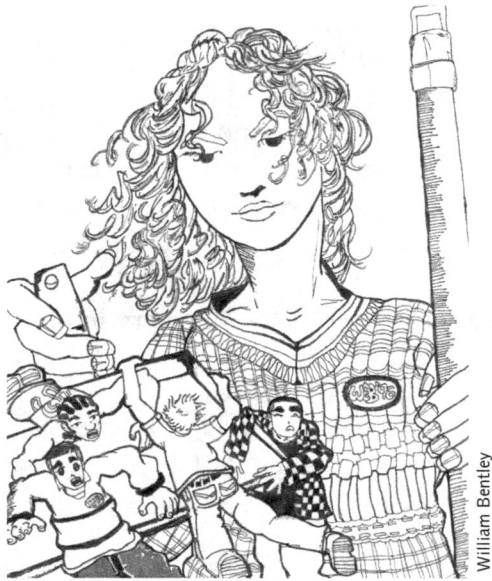

William Bentley

I Stopped Giving in to Him

By Anonymous

Most of my experiences with sex have had very little to do with love and care. I've been dogged out by guys more times than I care to remember. Even my current boyfriend has often seemed more interested in getting his nut off than in talking with me or holding me meaningfully. Normally I go along with it just to make him happy. But in the last few months I've been learning that if I want to get respect, first I have to respect myself.

When I was 14, I knew this guy named Shawn with soft and curly dark brown hair, and a light-brown chocolate complexion. He was 19, but he acted grown up, like he was 25. I wanted so badly for him to ask me to be his girl. I thought that going out with an older guy would make me look older, and then other older guys would notice me more.

One day Shawn and I were chilling in the attic of his house, drinking and smoking weed. We were sitting on a big soft couch in the dark watching television and he started to kiss me. The last thing I wanted to do was stop him; I thought he was starting to like me.

The next thing I knew, we were laying on the floor and Shawn said in a low voice, "I'm gonna put on a jimmy-hat, OK?" I just nodded my head and proceeded to take off my clothes. He went to the bathroom and stayed in there for what seemed like 15 minutes. "What's taking him so long?" I kept thinking.

When he finally came back, he still had his shirt on. "Let me see you," I asked suspiciously. I wanted to make sure that he really had on a condom. When he said no, in the back of my mind I was thinking, "Hold up, what's wrong with him?" but I was so drunk and high that I just went with the flow. It wasn't until about three weeks later, when I didn't get my period, that I found out Shawn hadn't had a condom on after all.

I was so scared that I kept my pregnancy hidden for about three and a half months. One time my sister was driving me to school, and I had morning sickness. Instead of telling her what was wrong, I just threw up in my mouth and swallowed the vomit back down.

My mother had a feeling that something was wrong with me, so she took me to her gynecologist. There, they found out for sure that I was pregnant and I decided to have an abortion.

Even after all that, I still wanted to be with Shawn (talk about being blind). The day after the abortion I went to his house. When I got there, he didn't even acknowledge the fact that we'd had sex together. "You know I was pregnant with your baby, right Shawn?" I said to him.

"Oh, word?" he asked without seeming to care. "What happened?"

I told him about the abortion, hoping that he would show me

a little compassion. "Oh," is all he said to me, like I was just one more girl that he had knocked up.

After Shawn, I got involved with a guy who used to punch me and curse at me. The only time that he was nice was when he wanted to have sex. I wouldn't leave him, though, because I didn't think I could do any better for myself.

After those and other bad experiences, it was hard for me to trust another guy. Then, last April, I met Duane, my present boyfriend. The week after I started at my new school, he just walked up to me and started a conversation. We went to the McDonald's by our school, and the whole time I was thinking, "He's just trying to hit it."

Duane confessed that he and two other schoolmates had bet who could bag me first (I guess Duane won).

Duane confessed to me that he and two other schoolmates had made a bet to see who could bag me first (I guess Duane won). Luckily for me he was being honest, because that told me to keep my eyes open and not to make myself vulnerable by falling in love with him.

After Duane told me about his little bet, it was even harder for me to believe that he wanted me for me. But I still gave him my number, and we started going out that day.

When we finally had sex, it was about a month into the relationship. I don't really enjoy sex that much. I was just doing it for Duane. We were in the basement of his house. I was so scared, because I didn't want Duane to tell all his boys in school that I let him hit the skins. "I hope you're for real," I remember telling him the whole time that we were having sex. "I don't want to get hurt again."

"I'm for real," he kept assuring me.

That first time Duane had asked me if I wanted to use a condom and I said yes. The next time we had sex, we didn't use one because neither of us had one. After that, if I brought it up he would try to manipulate me. One time he was kissing me seductively, and asked, "You want me to please you, right? If I can't feel you, how am I going to do that?"

I replied like I always did. "It's not about pleasing me," I said. "Because I don't get anything out of it anyway." The kissing didn't do anything to me, really, because sex doesn't faze me. But his groveling was a very pitiful sight. So, unfortunately, most of the time I just gave in.

The most annoying form of manipulation, though, was when he questioned my love for him. "If you loved me," he would tell me, "then you'd let me please you without a condom." Again, I would just give in.

I never really told Duane how I felt about unprotected sex or sex in general. The truth was, I hated the task of lying down knowing that I was going to do something tedious. Before I saw him I was always hoping he would just want to talk with me and find out what was on my mind. I would ask him for a condom before we had sex, but if he didn't have one we would do it anyway. That was that: No talk. No nothing. Just sex.

Lately, I've thought about the consequences that might result from unprotected sex, and I realize that taking care of my body is more important than making my man happy. I don't want anything more to happen as a result of my being irresponsible. I've already been pregnant twice. I'm not ready for a child now, and I worry that having another abortion could jeopardize the possibility of my having a family in the future.

But because I didn't communicate with Duane about how I felt, he never had a condom. On the other hand, neither did I. I always left it up to him. I thought it was his job even though I knew he didn't want to use one.

At the same time, the more Duane wanted to have sex without a condom, the more I believed that he just wanted me for my body. If I got pregnant, I figured he'd leave me.

One day after school, I went to his house like I usually did. Strangely, we were the only ones in the whole house that afternoon. As soon as he told me that we would have no interruption, I was disappointed. I knew what he had planned, and having sex was the last thing on my mind. I started watching television, to get him into something other than sex, but that didn't help. He started kissing my neck, and I was getting angry. I pushed him away first, and when he wouldn't stop, I told him, "Stop, I'm watching TV."

"C'mon," Duane told me. "Let's just do this before everyone comes home." That, I think, is what sent me over the edge. I got so pissed at him. It seemed as if he wanted me to do a "quickie" for him so that he could get his nut off. That proved to me that the only thing he wanted from me was sex.

That's when I finally spoke up about how I felt. I told Duane straight up, "I really don't like having sex with you, or anyone for that matter. It doesn't do anything for me, 'cause it's not what I care about at this time in my life. I have to finish school first, and then do what I feel is right for me."

I let him know everything that was on my mind. I confided in him about how I just went along with the sex mainly to please him. I assured him, however, that I loved him and that his manhood had nothing to do with it. It was just a question of what I wanted for myself at that time. Even so, he still felt the need to defend himself. "What, I'm not good enough for you?" he kept saying. "I can't satisfy you?"

After that conversation, Duane tried harder at pleasing me whenever we did have sex, and I started to feel hopeless about ever getting through to him. Every time he wanted to have sex and I didn't, either because he didn't have a condom or I just plain didn't want to, we would end up having sex anyway.

Duane thought that he had to satisfy me to keep me happy with him so I wouldn't have to look for pleasure anywhere else. If I said that I didn't want to have sex, and I was firm about it, then he would think that I was seeing someone else. He would also either pout or just go outside and not come back for the night.

He did that on two occasions. The second time I got so heated after he left me alone all night in his crib, worrying, that I screamed at him about the respect I deserve from him. After I gave Duane a piece of my mind, he realized that I wasn't joking around. Now he may be defiant once in a while, but overall, I've taken hold of our relationship.

Since I learned to communicate and to hold my ground, Duane now respects my wishes when I'm not in the mood. He also knows that if he doesn't have a condom then nothing sexual will happen between us. I've stopped giving in to his constant manipulating, and that has led him to stop trying to persuade me to do things I don't want to.

It isn't worth it to have unsatisfying sex just to please your boyfriend. After a while, you start to dread it.

I know, now, that if I don't want to have sex, then I don't have to. I will only truly enjoy sex if I do it when I'm ready. If my man can't handle that and he wants to leave, then it wasn't meant to be between us, and I still have time to find the right guy for me. It isn't worth it to have unsatisfying sex just to please your boyfriend. After a while, you start to dread doing it and can't make the sacrifice anymore.

Duane has grown up a lot, too. He understands that right now my education is the most important thing in my life and relationships are about walks in the park, long talks over the phone, communication (a biggie), and most importantly, love.

Personally, I think for sex to be enjoyable, both people have to be ready, know what they want, and feel the same way about each other. They have to care deeply and use protection. That way, no one gets hurt in the long run.

I know now that I wasn't ready for sex, and I don't know that

Am I Ready?

I ever will be. First, I need to get my priorities straight. My plan is to finish high school, start college, learn to depend on myself by living alone, getting a job, and living life to the fullest. But if I do things that I am not ready for now, then I won't be able to achieve these goals.

The author was in high school when she wrote this story.

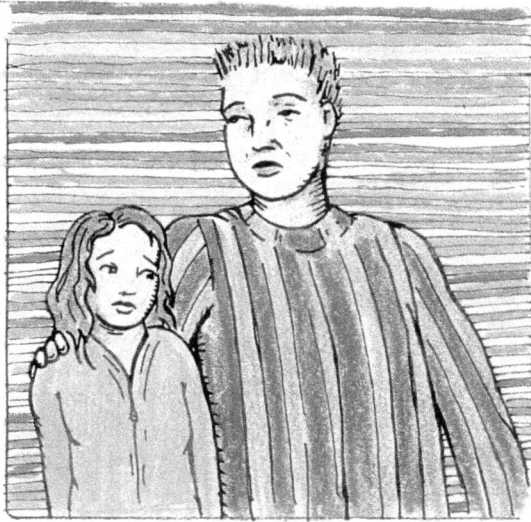

Shaun Shishido

When It Comes to Dating, Older Isn't Better

By Shaniece McKenzie

Let's talk about a dirty secret behind teen sex and pregnancy. You might think teenage boys are the ones getting girls pregnant. But research shows that many teen girls are being sexually exploited and impregnated by adult men, mostly men older than 20.

This is a major reality of teenage life that has been ignored. The same people who've expressed shock or concern about teens becoming mothers have not said much about the adults who have babies with babies. Now it is time to read the truth.

Several studies have found that adult men, age 20 and over, father anywhere from one-half to two-thirds of infants born to teenage girls in the United States.

And one California study found that men over 25 fathered twice as many babies as boys under 18. So it's not fair to blame teen boys for a lot of the teen girls getting pregnant. Also, many teen births are the result of sexual assault, according to the study.

Well, when I found all this out, I wanted to know more about why teenage girls go out with older guys. So I called the Youth Counseling League in New York City, and talked to a therapist named Gretta Mogel. Here's what I learned.

Mogel said girls who don't get emotional security at home may crave it, and older guys may give these girls the appearance of security. Girls who have been sexually abused are especially likely to look for relationships with older men.

Teenage boys and older guys both play a part in pressuring teenage girls to have sex. But unfortunately, young girls might trust an older guy more, even if that's not realistic. Teenage girls often feel that older guys will be responsible enough to take care of them if anything happens.

A girl should be aware of why older guys would fall for her. Older guys are looking at teenage girls for their innocence and youth. They may want to take care of them, or they may want to take charge. Never let a guy run your life!

Before entering a relationship with an older guy (or any relationship, for that matter), girls should think about the consequences the relationship could bring. A girl should know what she wants, and whether he wants the same thing. And she should know the history of his relationships.

Girls should also protect themselves from being emotionally hurt or taken advantage of, just as they would with a teenage boy. There are many risks that come with dating someone much older. Girls may feel like their boyfriends have everything and they have nothing. An older man generally has more power in the relationship than a teenage girl does, which can make the girl feel trapped, like she can never leave him.

Girls also have to decide whether to be open about the relationship. Teenage girls often have to hide the relationship from their family and friends. And, of course, you should know if he is married or has children. (You don't want to break up anyone's marriage, do you?)

Girls should also be extra careful and responsible with older guys, because girls have a higher risk of getting STDs and AIDS if they are having sexual relationships with adult male partners.

This is not to say that all relationships with older guys are bad. There are benefits (some older guys might actually be more responsible), and a girl may find someone who will treat her right. Still, she should keep this short list in mind:

Do:
Get to know him.
See if you can trust him.
Put your needs before his.

There is one big Don't:
Don't do anything you don't feel comfortable with, even if it means losing the relationship. (That's true for all relationships!) Girls, it's your body and you're in control.

*E*very state has laws against statutory rape to protect young girls from having sex with older guys under any circumstances, whether or not the girls give consent. (For example, in New York, a guy who is 21 or older cannot legally have sex with a girl who is younger than 17.)

You might be thinking: Wait a minute! Teenage girls aren't going to put the brakes on their hormones and postpone having sex just because it's decreed in law. So why do they even have these laws? The idea is that physically mature girls of 14 or 16 years old still have plenty of emotional growing to do, so they shouldn't be having sex with an older guy who could take advantage of them.

Laws aside, it's hard to know when you're ready. But even if the older guy you're dating pressures you to have sex, you need to decide for yourself.

Ms. Mogel said teenage girls may be physically and emotionally ready to have sex when they know how to take care of their bodies (like insisting on using protection!), know their morals, and won't feel guilty or angry at themselves afterward.

Still, by being with these older guys, I feel you're growing up too fast. It's OK to be a kid. And you know what, it's OK to be a virgin! If your boyfriend doesn't like that, he's not worth it. I know there's a lot of peer pressure out there, but it's not always right to follow the crowd. Just be yourself, because you're only a teenager once. Time stops for no one.

Girls who have been sexually abused are especially likely to look for relationships with older men.

My main advice is: Think about what you're doing. There are a lot of STDs out there. And you probably don't want to get pregnant, either. So keep it real with yourself, and think about what's right for you.

Shaniece was 15 when she wrote this story.
She went on to college at Lincoln University.

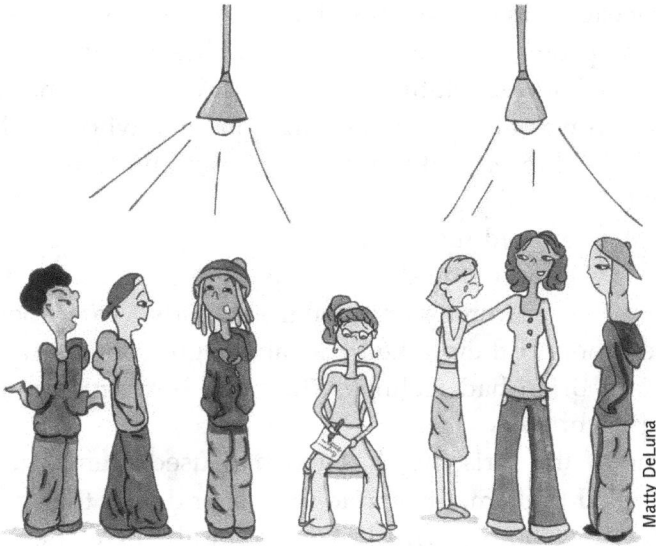

Matty DeLuna

Communication Is More Important Than Sex

By Anonymous

One day last July I was chillin' in the park with my three guy friends. As usual, I was the only girl there. We were playing cards when another girl walked by. "Yo. That girl over there looks mad good, but I heard she's mad easy," Mike blurted out.

"Excuse me, I'm sitting here," I said.

"And I'm just talking about some girl. That's just how I feel," Mike said. Then we all started talking about what had gone wrong in past relationships. This was a normal day in the park for Mike, Jamal, Brian, and me.

After a while, though, I started wondering why they said what they said about girls. I wanted to understand how guys saw relationships, so I started asking questions, like, "Why did you like her?" and, "What did you do after you broke up?"

They each told me how they handled relationships. Jamal just ended any problems by breaking up or cheating with a new girl. Mike never had luck dating, but he always tried to make things work. Brian was always looking for someone who could understand him. All three told me to be up front and to listen to what the guy had to say.

But they all told me what they really wanted was a girl they could relate to and would enjoy spending time with. I'd always heard that guys weren't emotional and didn't care about girls. But even though they talked bad about girls sometimes, Mike, Jamal, and Brian had feelings. They had been in love and had their hearts broken.

Some of the girls they'd dated had used them, cheated on them, or lied to them. I began to understand why they spoke the way they did about girls. I learned a lot about relationships by hanging out with my guy friends.

What I learned from my female friends, on the other hand, was nothing. The girls I knew thought that they had the upper hand in their relationships. But most of the time they were confused about what was going on. They were always getting dragged into some type of humiliation because they cared for a certain guy and thought that he felt the same way when he didn't.

My guy friends told me what they really wanted was a girl they could relate to and enjoy spending time with.

The girls would call me crying after they'd had sex and the guys had turned around and broken up with them. I'd listen, but most of the time I didn't really feel too bad for my girlfriends. I thought they were stupid to have sex so early, and I told them they'd be better off getting to know the guy first.

I noticed that girls and guys handled things in different ways. Girls I knew (including me at one point) just sat around and wondered what was wrong instead of asking. Guys tended to care but if the girls didn't ask questions, they pretended they didn't care. I think they should have stepped up and asked questions themselves. But I guess the guys I knew got tired of trying to make things work. With no real communication happening, they slowly gave up on the relationship.

Hanging out with both girls and guys helped me to see what can go wrong when you don't communicate. I wanted a relationship that meant something. It was important to me not to give myself emotionally and physically to a person who was just going to throw me away because he felt no connection and didn't know me.

I decided I wanted to date a guy for a while before having sex so we would know each other well. If he wanted to push the issue before I was ready, maybe that was all he was looking for.

Toward the end of the summer I started to like my friend Brian. He was smart and funny. When we all hung out together, he was quiet and usually did what I did—listen. When he spoke, instead of saying, "I dated this many people," like Jamal and Mike did, Brian would say things like, "This is the type of person that I was dating or want to be dating." Quantity wasn't important—quality was. He had the same values I had.

He asked me out a couple of times that summer and at first I was skeptical because I didn't want to ruin our friendship. But in September, I told him that I wanted to go out with him.

Soon after we started dating, we began to have conversations about sex and Brian would bring up the idea of us becoming intimate. Since I'd never had sex and he had, it was weird to talk about it. At first I'd just change the subject or pretend that I didn't hear what he was saying. I felt uneasy and I didn't want to end up like the girls I knew.

But one night, we were watching TV in his bedroom and I decided it was time to talk to him. Avoiding the situation wasn't helping me get my point across. In a single breath, I blurted out, "I care about you so much, but I don't want to do something that might end up ruining our relationship."

Having sex was still a big issue to me, I explained. I knew kids who were having sex and not being adults about it. To them, sex was just something you did because you were going out. I didn't see it like that. It got really silent and I felt nervous. I thought that maybe he wasn't going to respect my opinion. Brian got up and turned off the TV. Then he sat next to me and looked me in the eyes.

"Then I'm willing to wait until you feel comfortable enough with me to talk about it," he said. He reassured me that no matter what, he was still going to care about me and that sex wasn't a given. It was something special that took time to get to.

I felt relieved. In the past, I'd dated guys who had claimed that they knew we were going to have sex. They thought they deserved it because we were dating. But Brian didn't try to push it. He respected me enough to give me time to figure things out. I felt like I'd finally communicated what I wanted to him and he understood.

I work hard to know what's going on in my relationship, and it's worth the work.

After that, we continued to spend lots of time together and got to know each other even more, and our relationship grew. We argued, like most couples, but we also talked about how we felt and what we liked and didn't like. We spoke about sex and life and our relationship. Talking helped us understand each other and open up more about everything.

After a couple of months, we did decide we were both ready to have sex. It was nothing like the movies portray with roses and lit candles and everything. But it was special. We'd both invested lots of time getting to know each other first and we'd made the decision together. We had a deeper, closer relationship afterward and I felt like I had made the right decision.

We've been dating for almost a year and a half now and we have a real bond. Our relationship does have problems, but we try to work them out.

I'm glad that I didn't go along with my friends' ideas of what going out with someone meant—having sex and claiming the person as your boyfriend or girlfriend, but not actually communicating. I'm glad I took control of my own personal life and got the outcome that I wanted.

Mike and Jamal give us our space, but we still find time to hang out with them. They still talk about the girls who break their hearts and the girls they take advantage of. I still give them advice from time to time.

Brian still mostly listens, and sometimes he gives them advice based on how he and I get through our problems. He tells them to try to work through their differences with girls, and that if it doesn't work, maybe it wasn't meant to be.

Now when I listen to them talk, I'm happy to know that I don't have to deal with that boy drama. I can talk to my boyfriend and he talks to me. I work hard to know what's going on in my relationship, and it's worth the work.

The author was 17 when she wrote this story.

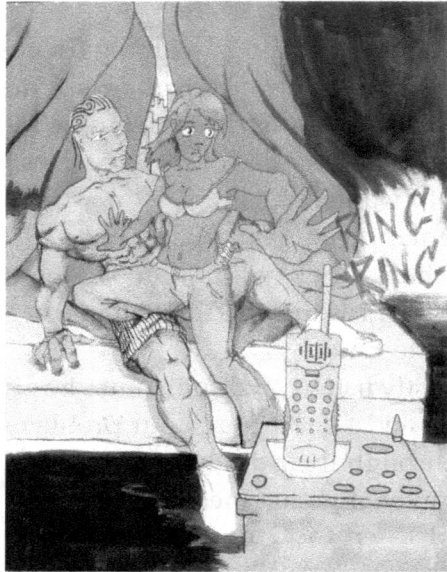

Gary Smith

Virgin Under Pressure

By Anonymous

I was excited when Jim asked me out last March. He'd tell me sweet things, like how he loved and cared about me and how good I looked, and how he wanted to see me every day. That made me feel like I was on top of the world.

I was also happy when Jim said that if I chose not to have sex with him, it was OK. "Finally, I met a guy who's into me but doesn't care if we have sex," I thought. It proved to me that he really cared about me.

I've dated about seven guys since I started high school two years ago. Not every guy I've gone out with pressured me to have sex, but it was the pushy guys I liked best, because they were the ones who gave me lots of compliments and told me how much they wanted to be with me.

It's OK with me if a guy I'm dating wants to have sex with

me because it makes me feel desirable. But I don't like it when they really pressure me. I'm not ready to have sex yet. Most of the pushy guys I dated broke up with me when I wouldn't have sex with them. With one guy I liked, that really hurt, because I felt attached to him.

But I feel I'm just not ready for the consequences of sex. I'm 16 and if I got pregnant, it would be a big disgrace to my family; my parents would beat me and kick me out of the house. I wouldn't want to abort if I got pregnant, but I don't want to be a teenage mother, either. I'm scared about catching an STI (sexually transmitted infection), too. I know that some STIs can cause infertility and there is no cure for HIV/AIDS.

When I'm not dating anyone, sometimes I feel like I'm ugly, or too fat, or just not good enough to make a guy like me.

But I think the biggest thing keeping me from saying yes to sex is that I'm not ready for the emotions. I would hate to have sex with someone and then have him leave me. That would be terrible—I'd feel used and thrown away.

Also, I have guy friends who talk badly about girls they have sex with, calling them whores or sluts. I don't want to be called that, or have people see me that way. I want people to see me as someone who knows how to control herself, who respects herself, who's smart.

But another part of me does want to have sex. Part of me thinks I would really like it. Movies, TV, music, books—they make it seem like sex is heaven. I can imagine that sex would feel wonderful if I feel like the person I'm with will love me forever and won't leave me—that the love we have between us is special.

Most of my friends have already had sex, and when they talk about it, I want to experience it, too. "It feels really good," one friend told me. "If you did it once, you'd want to do it all the time." For that second, I wanted to try it. But later I reminded myself that I'm waiting for a relationship that feels more sure, and that not having sex makes me feel special because I'm not like everyone else.

But Jim, who's 20, made me feel special, too. Not a day went by when we didn't see each other or talk on the phone. I liked being with someone who made me feel good about myself.

Often I feel insecure. When I'm not dating anyone, sometimes I feel like I'm ugly, or too fat, or just not good enough to make a guy like me. I compare myself to other people who I think are pretty or popular, and I feel very small.

It doesn't help when my friends or parents tell me I look nice. Then I feel it's just because they don't want to hurt my feelings. But when a guy tells me I look good, even if I think he's just sweet-talking me, I feel flattered. It makes me feel chosen.

Most of the time Jim and I talked on the phone because he was busy making money and I had to go to school. When he wasn't busy, he came to my house. We'd just hang out for about 15 minutes before kissing and stripping. It felt good.

I like having a boyfriend and being able to express the physical part of me. For me, being physical is tied up with emotions; it makes me feel more attached to the guy I'm with. I enjoy sexual behaviors like kissing, touching, and stripping—I just don't want to deal with the consequences of sexual intercourse. I know those behaviors can lead to sex, but I tell myself I can handle it.

With Jim, I had about a month before I had to start dealing with it. Even though he'd told me it was OK if we didn't have sex, it started to feel like when Jim was over, he was there to have sex with me. I noticed that he had condoms in his pocket. I started to worry about going too far. I was afraid that I'd get caught up in the moment and wouldn't say no.

Also, I thought that if I did say no to sex with Jim, he might get angry at me. I wanted him to be happy with me so he'd stay. I felt attached to him. He made me feel good about myself, and I didn't want to start over again getting acquainted with another guy. So I told him, "Maybe I will have sex with you one day, but not now." I wanted Jim to think he might have a chance to have sex with me so he'd stick around.

So instead of stopping myself, or stopping Jim when things started getting really sexual, I had my friends call me when Jim was over my house. In a past relationship, I'd discovered by accident that a ringing phone interrupts the moment and gives me a minute to think about what's going on. Then I stop whatever I'm doing and put my clothes back on.

But I wasn't sure how much longer I could keep putting off Jim—and sexual intercourse. Once, he pushed me on the bed for us to have sex. And since he was stronger than I was, I couldn't do anything about it. At first I thought he was just playing, but he kept pushing me down.

I realize that I didn't say anything to him directly about not wanting to have sex—I always made excuses.

He stopped, though, when I told him, "My mom is gonna be home very soon and you need to leave." I was relieved; his forcefulness had surprised me. I told myself that he should know that I wasn't ready to have sex with him.

But when I look back at it now, I realize that I didn't say anything to him directly about not wanting to have sex—I always made excuses, like my mom was going to come home, or that maybe I'd be ready one day, or I had my friends call me.

I was angry with Jim for pushing me down on the bed like that. But the next day, he called me at 8 a.m. and asked me how I was feeling. It made me think he still cared about me, and that reassured me. He didn't try to force me to do anything after that, but all we talked about on the phone was sex. He'd tell me how he couldn't wait to have sex with me and how he wanted to be my first.

If it made him happy to talk about sex, instead of actually having sex, that was fine with me. We could talk about sex all he wanted—I just didn't want to do it. But when he said things like,

"We're gonna have sex the next time I come to your house," I felt like I didn't want him to come over. I was afraid that he might actually try to have sex with me, and I didn't want to be in that situation. I felt flattered that Jim wanted to have sex with me, and I liked having Jim as a boyfriend, but I still didn't feel ready.

Over the summer, the pressure got more intense, to the point that I got scared to go to his house or for him to come to mine. Finally I told him outright, "I'm not ready to have sex," but he said that if I had sex with him I wouldn't regret it because it would be the best sex I would ever have.

I was confused. I remembered how he'd told me that it was OK if I didn't have sex with him and wondered what had changed. I felt that he was the one changing—but was he becoming the real him? I wouldn't have gone out with him if I'd known he was going to pressure me that much. But I couldn't bring myself to break up with him, either. I still liked the attention and thought I'd get lonely without him.

In August, he called and asked me to come over. Even though I felt unsure, I went because I wanted to please him. As soon as I walked in the living room, he started kissing me and taking off my clothes. Soon we were on his bed kissing, and he was touching me everywhere, which I enjoyed. Then I felt something trying to push in me, and he said, "Don't worry, I have a condom on."

I felt helpless and surprised. "Don't worry?" I thought. "Did I tell you that I wanted to have sex with you? If I wanted to have sex, it sure as hell wouldn't be with you." At that minute, I had no desire to have sex with him. I hated him. I told him, "Please get off me, please."

Then he asked me, "Are you scared?"

"Yes."

"Don't worry. If you want me to stop in the middle of it, I will." But as he was talking, he was trying to push his penis in me. I was trying to close my legs.

I thought, "Oh God, please let me leave this house still a

virgin, and if I get back to my house I will never step foot in this house again." I begged him to get off me and after a couple of seconds he did. I was so relieved. I just wanted to leave.

Jim got angry and called his cousins and told them he wanted to go out and they should pick him up. But as soon as he did that, I felt bad for not having sex with him, because he'd waited longer than most guys I dated and I wanted to make him happy and make him stay with me.

So when he asked me if I wanted to sleep next to him on the bed, I said yes. Even though he'd made me mad, I wanted to please him because I'd upset him by pushing him away.

So I put on my underwear and lay next to him, imagining he respected my decision to not have sex. I wanted to trust him because I wanted to believe that I could trust him. He started touching me again, which I didn't care about as long as he *I felt bad for not having sex with him, because he'd waited longer than most guys I dated.* didn't try to have sex with me again. But he did. As I tried to shove him off me, he kept trying to force himself on me.

This didn't feel like the sex that goes with love; I felt like he was trying to rape me. I was angry. I thought I'd made it clear that I didn't want to have sex, and he was still trying to do it. I shoved harder, and seconds later he got up, angry again.

This time I didn't care anymore if he was angry or not because I just wanted to leave. So I got up, put on my clothes and left him sitting on the bed. I still felt like I loved him, but I also felt very angry at him. I wondered if he'd break up with me since I didn't have sex with him. But at that moment, I didn't really care if he did. I trusted him less.

Over the next few weeks, I saw less of him. I began to suspect that I wasn't the only girl he was seeing. He wouldn't pick up the phone when I called him, and when I did talk to him, he gave me excuses about being busy that I didn't believe. That's what made me doubt that he still loved me. I felt stupid for being with him, and I hate feeling stupid. So I decided to stop going out with him.

A couple of weeks later, when I saw him standing outside with his friends, I went up to him and told him that I didn't want to go out with him any longer. It felt funny because I wasn't used to breaking up with guys. Usually they were the ones who broke up with me. But I felt proud of myself because I finally had the guts to end a relationship I wasn't happy with. I am still not sure about sex, but if I'm going to have sex with someone, I'd have to trust him more than I did when I first met him, not less.

I feel lonely without a boyfriend, especially when I have no one to call at night, but I don't want to go out with anyone for a while. My experience with Jim made me wonder why I wanted to please guys so badly, and why I didn't think about myself more.

I've started thinking, "What about me? What's wrong with me that I keep thinking about pleasing him? What about pleasing myself?" It made sense to me at the time, but now I don't know why pleasing a guy was so important to me.

So now I'm trying to figure out what I want. I'd like a long relationship. I don't want to see a boyfriend just once in a while. I want to spend a lot of time with him and do things together.

I think that what's best for me is to learn to be independent.

I'd like to be with someone who's confident. We can argue about things—that's OK, even fun sometimes, as long as no one gets really mad and curses. But I also want him to respect me and listen to me when I say I don't want to do something. And I want to be confident enough to tell a guy clearly that I'm not ready to have sex without being so afraid that he'll leave me.

It's hard to find guys who aren't so pushy around where I live. If I could find someone I like who likes me too, I think I could go out with him. But I think that what's best for me is to learn to be independent, and not care that my friends have boyfriends, or feel lonely because I don't have one. I want to stop comparing myself to others. It only makes me feel inadequate about myself, and that makes me vulnerable to guys when they flatter me.

I hope that when summer comes around again, I'll have learned my lesson and will feel happy being independent. I don't want another summer of pressure. Right now, I think my best option is not to have sex while I'm still in high school. I do want to have sex someday, but I want to do it with someone who respects me and who will be there for me for a long time.

The writer was in high school when she wrote this story.
She later graduated from college with a degree in psychology.

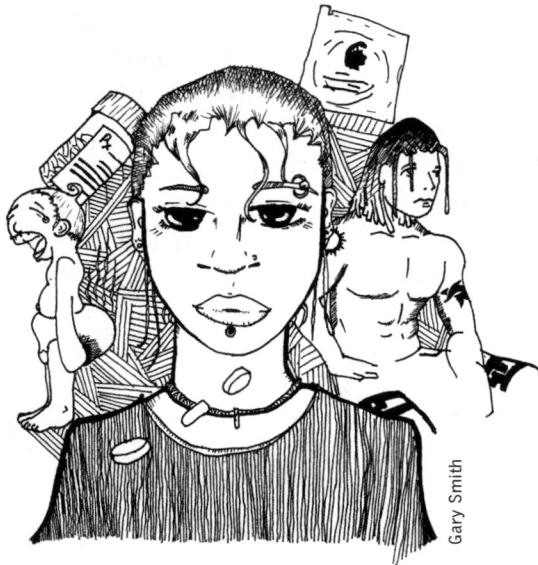

Gary Smith

The Morning After

By Anonymous

I'm a 20-year-old black female attending a university in the South. I first started having sex during my freshman year. I liked having casual sex, partly because I found on-campus relationships too complicated.

Recently I met a guy named Dante. He had decent looks and a good sense of humor. He was in the Army, majoring in civil engineering at a historically black college nearby. He took pride in being a black man doing big things, and that's very sexy to me.

I'd been seeing Dante for a couple of weeks when I called him over to my apartment on a Friday night during booty-call hours—any time between midnight and dawn. I supplied the liquor and he hooked up the movies. I had a few drinks because I was feeling so antsy. I was soon buzzed.

We finished one movie and then started to watch a second.

It felt like we were waiting to devour each other. We never finished watching the second movie. I was prepared for the moment when we started to get into each other, and had the condoms by the bedpost.

Only, that night, Dante had a hard time keeping his erection. We tried putting on the condom, but he shrank again. That's when I made the decision that I later came to regret: I decided to start having intercourse without a condom. I figured we could put on the condom after he was able to stay erect.

Granted, this is very risky behavior because of the presence of pre-cum, which is a liquid that comes out of the penis before ejaculation. Pre-cum can still carry infections like HIV and other STIs.

That night I decided to take a chance because I was less concerned about pre-cum than about having no sex at all. Dante maintained his arousal and then entered me. At this point, I thought to stop Dante and have him use a condom, but I didn't. I was buzzed and I also didn't want to break the rhythm we'd finally achieved. The night was finally taking off. I was caught up in the moment.

That is, until he let out an, "Oh damn!" We'd only been having sex for a few minutes. Dante pulled out and, with a look of mixed pleasure and fright, lay down beside me.

"I just came," he said, breathing heavily. I don't remember what he said after that because I was thinking, "I know you came quick. And possibly inside me." It seemed like he pulled out after he came, but I didn't ask him if he did because it felt like too hard of a question for me to ask.

"Could I get pregnant from this?" I wondered.

"Are you on birth control?" he asked.

"No," I said.

There was silence. I was determined not to panic. I wanted to wait until I was a little more sober and could sort everything out. So I went to sleep and let him spend the night.

With hugs and a kiss, we parted later that morning with an, "I'll be in touch." He sheepishly nodded and left. I knew I wasn't going to call him again.

I played the night's events back over in my mind. In my head were the excuses I'd heard from other girls who didn't think their risky behavior could get them pregnant: "It happened too quickly. He wasn't in long at all."

"Are you on birth control?" he asked. "No," I said.

I remembered sitting through the health lectures in high school and freshman year of college and the TV specials, thinking, "At this point, who doesn't know that unprotected sex can equal pregnancy or worse?" And here I was trying to convince myself that I couldn't be pregnant even though I'd just had unsafe sex!

I had homework to do, errands to run, and friends to catch up with, so I convinced myself not to worry. But I was two, maybe three weeks into my menstrual cycle, which is the time when women are most likely to get pregnant. Thoughts of my stupid actions and possible pregnancy seeped into my head in my apartment, at the food court, in the library, and in between friends' conversations.

I couldn't take a chance and wait to see if I was pregnant. I knew what I had to do. I would take the "morning after" pill—actually the "up-to-five-days-after" pill. One of my high school friends had a pregnancy scare a year ago and did a lot of research on emergency contraception (also called Plan B).

She told me how it worked. The sooner you take the pill the more likely it is to prevent pregnancy—and it's most effective within 72 hours (three days). The pill tricks your reproductive system into believing you're already pregnant. The body then builds a defense system to block a fertilized egg from settling in your uterus.

Even though I had a solution, I still wasn't clear about how to

handle it. And I needed to calm myself down. So Saturday afternoon I talked to my friend Sonya. We'd talked about birth control
before, so I thought she could soothe my anxieties by giving me
informed advice and not judging me.

Still, Sonya's eyes bugged out and her mouth fell open when I
told her I'd let Dante hit it raw. She told me that I could possibly
be pregnant; she said the best thing to do would be to go to the
school's clinic on Monday and talk with a professional about getting the morning after pill.

But it was only Saturday and I worried about waiting two
days. The more I tried to push negative thoughts out of my mind,
the more they pushed back. I didn't want to wait things out and
see if I turned up pregnant. I'd assumed that if I had an unwanted
pregnancy, I would have an abortion. But now that the possibility
seemed real, I worried I would consider abortion murder. On the
other hand, I had no desire to be anyone's mother. Having a child
would wreck my chances of achieving my goals.

My worry was like a little snowball that got bigger and bigger as it rolled down the hills of my mind. I spent the rest of
the weekend doing homework,
waiting, worrying. I just wanted
to get to Monday, get my pill,
and move on.

*I let my desire for good sex get
the better of me.*

At 8:30 Monday morning, I
made an appointment over the phone with the student clinic to
get the morning after pill. A million thoughts passed through my
mind in the hour between the call and my appointment.

"Should I tell Dante what I'm doing?" I wondered. "And
could I tell my mom?"

"No," I told myself. If I took the pill, I wouldn't get pregnant.
I wouldn't tell Dante because we hadn't been a couple and didn't
have a major emotional attachment. He hadn't even called to see
if I was OK.

As for mom, I wanted her to think that I was safe. From this point on I knew I would be and didn't see any reason to upset her. It would be hard for me to forgive myself for disappointing her.

At the clinic, a nurse saw me first. While taking my temperature and blood pressure, she asked me if the sex was consensual, if I'd failed to use a condom or if it had broken, and if I was on birth control. I said the sex was consensual. A few minutes later, Dr. M. entered.

Dr. M. asked me the same questions and recited information about the importance of consistently using condoms and the need to protect myself against sexually transmitted infections. Dr. M. said I should use birth control if I couldn't be counted on to use condoms regularly. As she talked, Dr. M. bobbed her head back and forth with the authority of a judge with her gavel. Then she said, "If you keep this up, it's only a matter of time before you get pregnant."

I felt stupid having to listen to her speech. I hated feeling like I was a stereotype, one of too many black girls who can't remember to use condoms and end up pregnant.

Dr. M. gave me the first of the pills right there in her office with instructions to take the next one in 12 hours. I took the last pill at 9:30 that night in the library, well on my way into studying all night.

They were the smallest pills in the world, but they felt larger than the vitamin horse pills I take daily. I felt hopeful that the worst was over when I swallowed the pill and said, "Now do your thing." Luckily, I didn't suffer any physical side effects from the pills. There could've been nausea, vomiting, vaginal spotting, and headaches.

My pregnancy problem was over, but I still had a lot of questions. Over the next few days, I tortured myself with conflicting thoughts about sex and relationships, and wondered if I'd ever be tempted to not use condoms again.

And I questioned if I should just have serious relationships and give up booty calls. What hit me hardest about the experience was that I let my desire for good sex get the better of me. Instead of putting off sex when things weren't working, I got caught up in the heat of the moment.

I still feel that sex is a beautiful thing; my desire's normal and won't shake. But I can control the situations in which I have sex so I don't do foolish things. I don't ever want a nightmare like the one I had over not using condoms.

Dante called me about a month after my pill drama. He talked to me like nothing had happened. I told him that I had to take emergency contraception. He sounded relieved that I wasn't pregnant. Then he admitted that he came inside me. Hearing him say that made me realize he didn't deserve me. I was right about my decision to take responsibility for myself.

My new partner's more considerate. We've had sex a couple times and he's as insistent about using condoms as I've become. Like me, he's scared of pregnancy and infections and wants to maintain his peace of mind. Looking back to that weekend with Dante, I was too antsy about having sex with him. Now I take time to enjoy the moment and remember to be safe.

The author was 19 when she wrote this story. She earned a bachelor's degree in economics and went to law school.

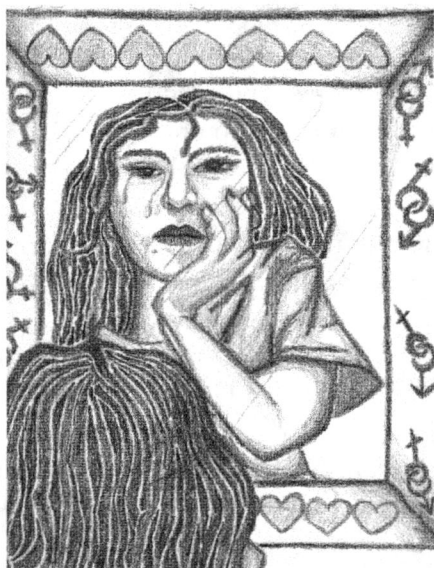

Elizabeth Deegan

Looking for Love

By Fetima P.

My boyfriend had always known about my past, but one day toward the beginning of our relationship, he asked me how many guys I'd had sex with. "A lot," I said. But he wanted a specific number. I was shocked when I counted and realized the answer was 21. That even shocked him. So then I asked him the same question, and when he answered, I was speechless for the first time in my life. He said, "One."

I don't think I've ever felt so bad in my life. Not even when people called me names did I ever feel that bad. When I came out of shock, I burst into tears. He told me I shouldn't be upset—I really am a nice girl who didn't know what she wanted from a man, he said. Actually, I did know what I wanted from a man— the problem was, I didn't know how to get it. I wanted someone who would give me all the love and support I didn't get at home.

What I got instead was just sex.

I guess I figured that if I could find a nice guy to treat me right, he would automatically take the place of my father, who left home when I was in the 6th grade. I was very hurt when my father left because we had such a good relationship. We would go to Florida by ourselves for the weekend and leave my mother home. We'd go out to dinner and to the movies. And it meant a lot to me that (and this may sound silly) we even had special names for each other. If we had such a good relationship, why was he leaving me? What had I done wrong?

After my father left, I was upset and depressed, and I began to rebel against my mother. I felt like I couldn't depend on her for the love I needed because she's not very open. She says I can talk to her, but I don't think I can. I didn't know any other way to vent my feelings, so I would keep all my anger inside and wait until she got me upset. Then I'd go off on her. I always wanted to tell her my problems and tell her what I was doing with my life, but it seemed like the older I got, the harder it was for me to tell her anything. I felt like my life was one big secret.

I wanted someone who would give me all the love and support I didn't get at home.

After my dad left, I also shrugged off all my girl friends. I felt like they couldn't do anything for me except tell me where the cute guys were going to be. They couldn't help me with my real problems. I felt like I had no one to talk to and I didn't feel close to anyone. I started to feel empty inside.

I only knew one way to fill that empty space, and that was to depend on a guy emotionally the way that I used to depend on my father. I was 12 ½ years old when my father left, and by my 13th birthday, I had lost my virginity. Afterwards, I wasn't proud of it, but how could I change it? It was already gone.

The first time I had sex was the biggest surprise of my life. At the time, I was mad at my boyfriend and wanted to get back at him. Another boy took me to a friend's house and we had sex in his brother's room. I had no intention of doing that. I went to our friend's house as the most naive virgin in the world, honestly thinking that nothing would happen if we were alone. Later I found out we weren't even alone: There was one guy watching from under the bed and another guy watching from the next room.

Once it was all over and the audience was gone, I didn't even know how to feel. But I didn't feel bad until I found out that the guy under the bed wanted to know if he was next.

When I got home, I went into my room and wrote in my diary. That's when it really hit me. I thought to myself, "Fetima, you just had sex with someone who doesn't even love you!" I sat there and cried. To make things worse, the guy broke up with me two days later.

I didn't have sex again for a while. I figured I wouldn't want to do it again. But when the urge did arise, I didn't fight it. I made out with all these guys who came my way, and my name was scattered all over my neighborhood.

I was 12 ½ years old when my father left, and by my 13th birthday, I had lost my virginity.

I never really felt that I had to go all the way with them, but that's the way it happened. I had this I-don't-care attitude, but I did care even though I wouldn't admit it. I would cry every night thinking about what I was doing and how I felt. Still, I couldn't seem to change. I always wondered to myself, "What the hell is your problem? Don't you know you could catch something and die?"

I never had an answer for any of the questions that I asked myself. I felt like a lost soul walking through a graveyard, trying to find someone to take care of me, but never picking the right one. I would always go into the bedroom thinking this guy might actually like me. Then when we finished and everyone knew about it the next day, I would realize I was wrong again.

But again and again my feelings would get intertwined way too much. I'd get a big knot in my chest and think it was love. Then I would get upset with the guys when they didn't return my feelings, even though I knew deep down inside that they hardly even knew me. And the truth is that I really didn't know them either.

It's not so much that I thought that sex would lead to love, but I guess that as a girl, I thought everyone felt close after they had sex. Ten times out of 10, though, I ended up being the only one who felt something at the end of the night. I guess I just had to learn the hard way that some guys will tell you anything to keep you in their houses a little while longer.

Most people who found out what I was doing labeled me a "ho" and a "slut." They never tried to find out what was wrong, and just assumed I was doing this for the fun of it. But I never enjoyed myself. I mean, I enjoy having sex whether I like the sex or not, but mostly because I enjoy pleasing the person I'm with.

I don't know why I feel I have to satisfy other people all the time. I don't want to hurt anyone's feelings and I'm afraid they might think less of me if I don't do what they want me to do. I tend not to tell people what I truly feel. I usually just say what the person wants to hear.

For example, I was going out with a guy who made it clear he just wanted me for sex. One day I didn't feel like being bothered, but I also didn't feel like I could tell him I didn't want to have sex. So while he was in the bathroom, I just took my stuff and left. The next day I saw him driving by as I was walking home from work. He stopped the car in the middle of the street and yelled at me and called me names.

My experience with that guy made me look at my other relationships. I said to myself, "Fetima, you're so stupid!" If I'd had two other hands, I would have beat myself up.

I never knew just how bad I felt about myself until a good

male friend of mine wrote me a letter telling me it was high time I took a look in the mirror and saw that I was not the person I was acting like. When I read his letter, I started to cry. I had never really thought I was a ho or a slut, because I always wanted to stay in school and make something of myself. I thought that made me different. My friend's letter made me see that I was acting like a slut, even though I knew I was worth more than that.

The person who really helped me calm down is my current boyfriend. He and I have been together for almost three years now, even though we've argued, cheated on each other, and even broken up during that time. He has helped me realize who I am and who I want to be.

I didn't have sex with him for a whole year, as a kind of test to see if he'd wait—and he did. He wanted a serious, not just a sexual, relationship. That made me feel more confident in myself. Now I can proudly say that while I haven't made a 180 degree turnaround in my life, I have made a 90. I'm really proud of myself for that. Some people can't even make a 9 degree turn.

In the same time that it takes to call someone a slut or a ho, you could talk to her.

These days, I am still flirty and I still feel like having sex with some guys I meet (and sometimes I do). But I'm working on being monogamous. When I tell guys no, I feel proud of myself. To myself, I'm like, "You go, girl!"

I always tell younger girls that I wish I had never had sex in the first place. I know that if someone had told me that, I probably would have gone and tried it anyway. But I think it's important for girls to know that having sex with every guy, or even a select few, isn't cool. In my opinion, there is nothing wrong with having responsible sex, but if you don't want to have sex, or you don't enjoy having sex, you shouldn't do it.

Plus, sex is risky. Of course, you can get pregnant. And there are millions of people out there with AIDS and other diseases. We teenagers think that it's never going to happen to us. But it does!

If you're the type to call a girl names and make her feel bad—well, take it from someone who has been there, it hurts like hell. In the same time that it takes to call someone a slut or a whore, you could take some time out to talk to her. Ask her why she chooses to do the things that she does. She may be surprised at first by your asking, but I bet she will be happy that you cared enough to ask.

Fetima was 18 when she wrote this story.
She had a daughter when she was 19.

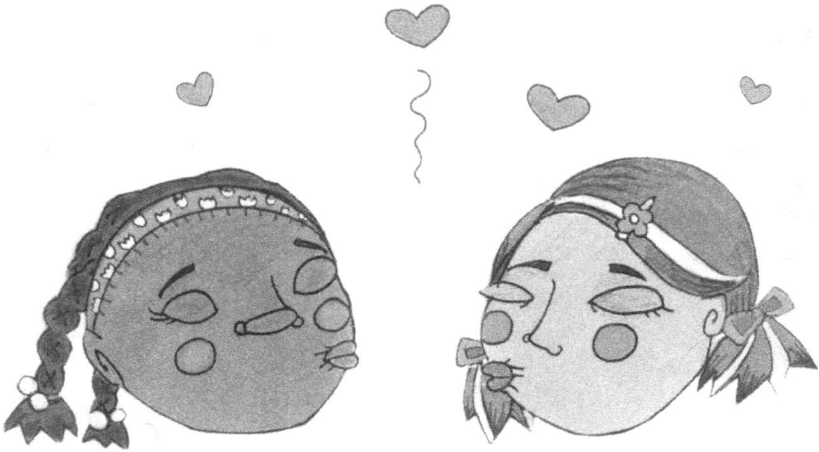

Karolina Zaniesienko

I Need a Girl

By Destiny

I was a 13-year-old high school freshman when I realized that I was attracted to females. I felt funny because I didn't know anyone who was a lesbian. I didn't understand why I was feeling this way, so I wasn't comfortable with my attraction. I didn't want to face that I was seriously looking at girls like a guy would.

I didn't think I could reveal my attractions to any of my friends, because, for us, it was about how to get boys to like you. I'd had "boyfriends" and had even kissed a boy. So I convinced myself that I was merely curious about being with the same sex.

But one girl brought a major change to how I looked at my sexuality. She lived near my house. I usually saw her around, often by the neighborhood church. But I didn't know her name. Every time I saw her, I stared and got nervous and clumsy. My heart beat like a drum and my chest got tight. I even tripped on the curb once while looking at her walk.

One day I was with my friend Susan and we saw her again.

"Hi Keesha," Susan said.

"Wassup, girl," Keesha replied. Susan introduced me to Keesha, and we said right there that we should hang out since we saw each other so often.

I started to spend a lot of time with Keesha on the weekends and saw her after school sometimes. We were the same age and both liked to watch horror movies and write. Sometimes we acted out our stories at home. And when we went shopping together, we bought each other gifts.

I convinced myself that I was merely curious about being with the same sex.

Spending time with Keesha made me like her a lot more. About two months after we were introduced, I decided that I had to tell her how I felt about her. I knew it was risky but I couldn't hold it in any longer. I was scared that my feelings for her would get too intense if I continued to hold them in.

We were at her house one day, and I knew I had to tell her then and there. My palms were sweating and my head started to itch. I had no idea what she'd tell me after I told her. Keesha had acceped that her mother's bisexual and that her best friend, Michael, is gay. Still, I didn't know how she felt about a girl having feelings for her.

So, as we were gossiping, I came out and said, "I have to tell you something."

"What?" she replied.

I stalled, and then said, "Well, before I met you, I used to see you all the time."

"You used to look at me mad funny," she said.

"Well... I was just looking because I was attracted to you," I said timidly.

Keesha looked very surprised. Then she blushed. "Well," she said. "I like you too."

Am I Ready?

This could not be real. I kept on asking her if she was serious. Although she kept saying yes, it didn't hit me until she kissed me on my lips. I'd never kissed a girl before. When I'd kissed a boy, I felt nothing. When I kissed Keesha, I felt butterflies in my stomach. Her lips felt like rose petals and tasted like orange lip gloss.

After we got over the initial shock of our attraction to each other, Keesha and I became a couple. But we never showed it in public. We always made sure that whoever saw us thought of us as friends. We weren't ready to be criticized by other people, so we told no one about our romance.

What mattered more to me was that Keesha was in my life. I cared for Keesha a lot and hugged her tight every time we met. I wrote her letters almost every day. We spent hours talking on the phone and texting each other.

About a month and a half into our relationship, she told me she loved me. And I loved her too. My time with Keesha made me realize how happy I could be dating a girl. I loved it. Before meeting her I daydreamed about being with a girl and being happy, and being with Keesha was even better than I'd hoped.

Keesha's lips felt like rose petals and tasted like orange lip gloss.

Unfortunately, my relationship with Keesha started to change soon after we revealed our love to each other. I started going to dance practice on Saturdays and after-school classes, so I saw her less. She started to put on a musical for her school and to sing in the talent show.

We stopped having time for each other. One night on the phone I told Keesha we were drifting apart. I said we should just be friends. She sounded sad. I felt sad too. I cried after I hung up because I didn't want her to hear me cry and then start crying herself. It was hard, but I felt it was for the best.

My relationship with Keesha lasted three months. Thankfully, we're still friends. Soon after being with her, I made up my mind that I was a lesbian and that I didn't want to be with guys anymore. The strong love and attraction I felt for Keesha was what I knew I could feel for another girl, not a guy.

Three months after breaking up with Keesha, I started to tell some of my friends I was a lesbian because I felt comfortable enough with my sexuality to risk coming out. I also told my parents.

I'm 16 now and have dated other girls since Keesha. Some of those relationships have been even better than when I dated her because they were out in the open.

I have a girlfriend now. I can hold her hand in public and not care about the eyes that I know are looking at us. I can kiss her in public without looking over my shoulder to see if anyone I know is around.

My relationship with Keesha helped me get to this point. She was my first girlfriend, and I'll never forget her.

The author was in high school when she wrote this story; she went on to college.

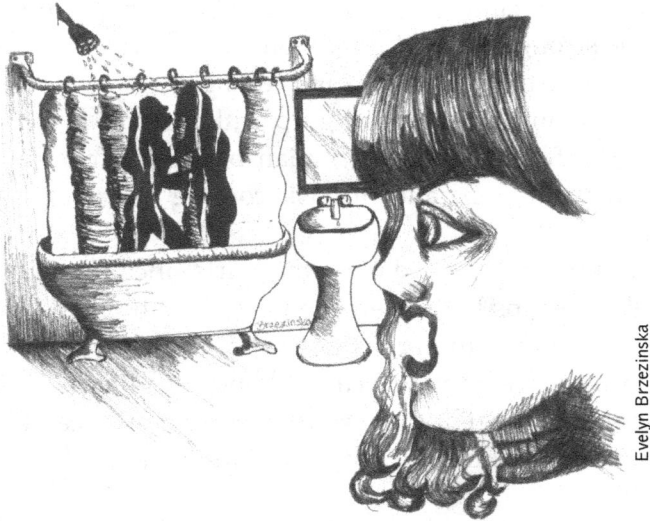

All Men Are Dawgs

By Wunika Hicks

Have you ever had a man who spoke sweet nothings in your ear, saying how beautiful you were and how much he loved you, and that you were the only one? And in return you blushed, giving him your heart and time, only to get played? Well, my dear, that kind of man is a dawg.

Now, a lot of men say that they aren't dogs, but it's either because they're on the low (gamin'), they've reformed themselves (let's assume for the better), or they don't even know (slow). But they either was a dog, is a dog, or too stupid to even know that they are a dog.

One day I went to my boyfriend Shawn's house to surprise him. His 8-year-old brother let me in. Honey, I went into Shawn's room in the basement and there he was in the shower with some girl, tellin' her how soft she felt in the water.

60

What could I do? (I know what I should, would, and could do now, but that's something different!) I just went quietly up the basement steps, feeling the hurt and pain of having my trust betrayed by a guy who I believed to be true.

Shawn tried to conversate on the telephone about two days later, talking about how much he missed seeing my pretty face and how he wanted me to come by his house that night. I couldn't even bring up what I had seen two days before. I just acted like I wasn't interested every time he called, until he finally dumped me.

Now, don't get me wrong—just because you date more than one female at a time doesn't make you a dog. It's all about honesty.

Just because you date more than one female at a time doesn't make you a dog. It's all about honesty.

one female at a time doesn't make you a dog. It's all about honesty. If you can tell a lady up front that you're dating other people and she still wants to get into a relationship, then what's so bad about that?

I dated a guy named Andy who told me he had a girlfriend, but I still decided to date him. One day I went to his house (this time by appointment) and we were talking about his relationship with that chick.

Well, honey, didn't you know that during the conversation he said that he and his wife were having problems. I said, "WIFE?!" You know I was buggin'.

He tried to cover it up by saying; "Oh, didn't I tell you about my wife?" (You see, Andy had a combination of the dog. He was gamin', and he was doing it on the low, but he was also stupid because he was slow!)

I couldn't do nothing but look at him in awe, while Andy continuously asked me, "What's the matter?" WHAT WAS THE MATTER!? I was through.

Why can't men just be real about their intentions? Why must they sleep with this chicken (that's what they call females) and that chicken, and gas up this one to get her on their lists to show off and brag, while they receive pounds over how many they've accumulated in the last hour?

I know you men and some women are saying: "Some women dogs, too. It's not just men." I disagree, because there are a lot of things that men can do and get credit for that females can't, even though they're capable, and being a dawg is one of them!

For example, there's this girl who lives in my neighborhood named Kizzy. Every day she has a new man on her shoulder, and even though no one knows what she does with them behind closed doors, guys look at her as just another girl to try and knock up. Because what do they have to lose? Their virginity? Please!

One day I went walking into my neighborhood store and Kizzy happened to be there. There were a bunch of guys on line and they were eyeing her. As soon as she left, they said:

"Damn, that b-tch's body is a dime, her face ain't all that, but I'd still hit that to see if what my man John said was true."

Why? Why can't Kizzy just do whatever she does and be left alone? Why must she be judged and put through humiliation just because she has more than one male friend? Why can't a woman be a dog with all the props that men get?

Why is a woman judged and put through humiliation just because she has more than one male friend?

As you noticed, the guys in the store called Kizzy a b-tch and yes, that does mean female dog, but it's used in a different context. The way I define dog is a man who does nothing but game, a man who's not straight up.

But those males who talked about Kizzy and called her a b-tch were really reversing it, because they were the ones who were trying to use her instead of it being the other way around.

And instead of Kizzy getting pounds for having a lot of boyfriends, women look at her in disgust. Why? Kizzy doesn't have any of their men on her shoulder, yet she gets looked down upon. I say it's just jealousy, because they see a female who they assume is doing something that men have been doing for years—playing the field. They are so used to a man playing girls in the open or on the low that when they see a lady doing it, they think:

"Oh, I can't believe her, she is actually playing all of those men. That is so wrong. I can't wait until one of them catches her."

A woman can play her game on the low, she can be reformed for the better and not for worse, or she can be a little slow and do it and not even know, but she'll never be considered a dog.

No, it's more likely she'll be considered a ho. That's because in this world, when it comes to sex, whatever a woman does— good or bad—she can never be equal to a man!

Wunika was 18 when she wrote this story.
She later went to college.

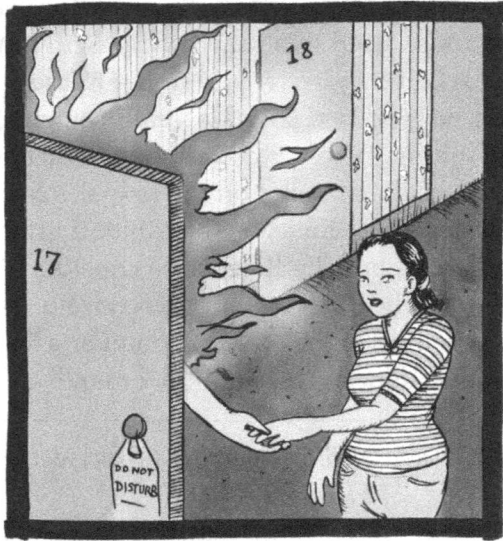

Shaun Shishido

I Was Scared but
I Wanted Experience

By Anonymous

When I was 16, my friends Sasha, Jasmine, and I made a bet over who'd lose her virginity first. We were the last holdouts in our larger group of friends. Several of my friends said they'd been having sex since they were 14, and Kelly proudly said she'd started even younger. I wasn't sure I believed them, but I thought a lot about what they said.

I mainly thought they were too young to be having sex. Only recently, it seemed, we were playing with Barbie dolls, and now they were talking about all the sexual things they did and what they wanted to try out next. As for myself, I often felt like a little girl lost in a grown woman's body.

Growing up, I didn't want to have sex. Until I was 15, I wanted to be a nun: sacred and untouchable. Then I started to live in this magical world where I could be married and have kids but still be a virgin. I was terrified of having sex. I heard things from my friends, like, "The first couple of times, it hurts and you bleed."

Me, pain, and blood don't mix. And I couldn't think about having sex without feeling guilty for going behind my parents' backs. If they found out, I thought, they'd scream and yell at me because I was too young to be having sex; it wasn't acceptable according to my family's traditional values.

I'd heard my mother say how kids are getting wilder, hornier, and dumber, particularly ones around my way. Those were the kinds of kids that my family and people I admired looked at with disgust. I didn't want to be that.

It wasn't just sex that I was afraid of, though. Serious relationships scared me too, because I didn't want to get hurt. I remember desperate-sounding girls calling my house crying after my brother broke up with them. He'd make me answer their calls and put them on speaker phone; then he made fun of them after they hung up. I didn't want to be humiliated like that.

Just worrying that the guy I liked wouldn't like my friends, or vice versa, was enough to keep me from attempting a relationship. Plus the idea of having sex with a guy who I really cared for scared me; I was afraid of having that beautiful feeling, and then having it drop down to the ground just as easily as it went up.

Still, I was the oldest one among my friends, and to hear them talk about having sex made me feel like I was younger than they were. I told myself, "If they can do it, why can't you?" But then I'd think, "You're too young. Don't you want to wait until marriage? It'll be more romantic."

I'd go back and forth in my mind:

"There's so many people in the world; do you really think you're going to stay with one guy forever? Don't you want to see how other guys are?"

"That's how diseases spread."

"I'm not dumb."

"You are if you're thinking about having sex just to get it over with."

A couple of months before the bet, my friends and I had adopted a new phrase—"It's all for experience"—which I came up with because I wanted some adventure in my life. I heard a lot of people say the best way to learn is from experience, which I believe. So even though I was scared of sex, I entered the bet.

Having sex just for the experience seemed easier than trying to get into a relationship in order to have sex. I thought that maybe I could detach myself from the emotional part of sex so I wouldn't get hurt if we broke up.

My curiosity grew, but I didn't have much opportunity to have sex. The guys around my way? Hell no! They were my brother's friends and way older than me. My brother told me to stay away from them. And that was fine with me because they were the type of guys my mother looked at with disgust.

As for the few guys I had crushes on, I tried to avoid them because I was scared they wouldn't understand me or like me. But my friends were getting action and I felt left out. Besides, I was having problems at school and at home. I was depressed and longed to get rid of that feeling. I thought sex might help.

So during Christmas vacation, a few weeks after the bet, I decided to go for it with Ralph. I'd known Ralph for two years. He was a year younger than I was and (from what he and his friends said) had already had sex when he was 14.

He'd wanted a relationship with me since the year before. I'd considered going out with him, since he was cute, and he wasn't a "playa," but he did dumb things like stand on the fire escape ripping up paper and yelling "Parade!" I thought I should at least respect the guy I'm with, but I also thought he was as good as I was going to get.

I told Ralph to come over to my house at noon and called my friend Sasha and told her to come at exactly 1 p.m., so I'd have an escape in case I decided I didn't want to go through with having sex.

I told Ralph to bring the condom, "just in case." We started kissing, which was nice because he tasted like Snickers. But kissing was as far as I'd ever gone with a guy, and the idea of going from kissing straight to the boogety-woogety felt so freakin' weird. My mind wasn't feelin' it, so neither was my body.

I held off as long as I could, but then things started heating up—our pants were down and Mr. Wiggles needed a jacket. I was thinking, "When is he going to pull out the condom, and when the hell is Sasha going to come?" And that's when I was saved by the bell. Sasha knocked loudly on my apartment door, scaring Ralph off me.

I felt so relieved. But I was also slightly disappointed because I had the chance and didn't take it. Sasha and I pretended that we were in a rush to go somewhere. I gave Ralph a kiss goodbye and we all left.

I felt like an idiot. I was just a kid, wishing to be grown-up by having sex. Plus, I didn't think it was fair to use Ralph like that, even though he knew about the bet and said he was fine with it.

After that, we only spoke three more times on the phone, and then we never talked again. I didn't want to see his face anymore because there'd always be that "almost-event" on our minds. And I didn't want to remember it because I felt so stupid. I decided to take things slower from then on.

But a year later, when I was 17, I got a second chance.

I met Chris in a hotel hallway in Georgia, at a friend's 21st birthday. As I walked my friend Kim to the elevator, she stopped Chris in the hallway and said, "Hey! Boy, doesn't she look fine?"

"Boy?!" said Chris. "I ain't no boy."

Kim looked at him and giggled, "You know what I mean... son!"

Chris smiled and said, "Yeah, she looks cute." I blushed and they started teasing me. Then Kim got in the elevator and Chris and I stayed.

I thought he was charming and cute—a beautiful smile, with dimples—and he was 6 feet tall, and built. We talked for nearly two hours in the hallway about almost everything, including… sex. I even told him I was a virgin and that I would only do it with someone I loved. (I guess I sorta stretched the truth.)

He told me about his sexual experiences, including details I didn't need to know but was curious enough to ask about. He was three years older than I was, and wasn't a virgin.

I didn't want people to keep looking at us, since it was so obvious that he was trying to talk to me, so I finally let him into my room. I suspected something big was going to happen. What happened next was all a blur. I didn't understand why I didn't stop. But it wasn't like I wanted to stop either, because I was curious and thinking to myself, "It's all for experience." He closed the door, turned the TV way up, and things went on from there.

Afterwards, he looked at me and smiled. I wanted to punch him in the face.

In the beginning, it was lovely; we were just kissing. The kissing was fun, the caressing was nice, sweet and romantic, but the initial you-know-what wasn't. Painful? Hell yeah!

We used a condom. I wouldn't have done it if he didn't have one, since I wasn't into catching an STD or getting pregnant. So many things were happening at once and I felt a wave of emotions: "OH MY GOD, wake me up! Why am I here? I'm actually doing it. I want to call my friend. Is this how it's supposed to feel? I want to go home. I want him to love me." I knew that I'd changed, but didn't understand how.

Afterwards, he looked at me and smiled. I wanted to punch him in the face. I didn't feel good about it. It felt like a wrong move. I rationalized to myself that everyone else on the floor was having sex, but that didn't make me feel better. I felt like a grownup because I'd had sex, but a stupid one. I felt like a fool because I was with someone who was practically a stranger.

I wondered if it would have felt the same if I were with some-one I knew and loved. I hadn't felt any real passion. And what was I going to do when I got home? Would I tell my mother? Could she find out just by looking at my face? Should I tell Kim and Sasha or keep it to myself?

"So what's up? Talk to me," he said.

I didn't want to talk to him. I didn't want to look at him. I hated him. I turned over and said that I was sleepy. I pretended to sleep, but I was thinking about the whole thing. I wanted to cry. I thought I had more respect for myself than to just do it with a stranger. Was he the slut or me?

Chris stayed in my room until 5 a.m., because we all had to leave by 7 a.m. to take the plane home. I went into the shower hoping to wash off the feeling of failure. He tried to talk to me during the bus ride to the airport and on the plane, but I ignored him and sat with other people.

But I'd given him my number before we'd started fooling around, and once we got home, he called me persistently. I thought it was sweet the first time he called, but then I thought he was just being nice to me because he felt guilty, and I didn't want any of his sympathy.

I was afraid to let myself feel romantic toward him, because then I'd be emotionally vulnerable. I didn't think that he genuinely liked me. Because he was older, I thought he could have any woman, and would probably prefer ones his age.

I was still all shook up from the things I remembered doing. I worried that he just wanted to do it again. I didn't want to feel like I was being used for sex. I was so focused on the fact that I'd had sex, I was blind to the clues that he actually liked me, like his frequent friendly calls. I just thought, "God, why doesn't this punk stop calling me?!"

Even my mother noticed I wasn't acting like myself. I was unusually quiet and wrote nonstop in my journal, recording every thought I had, trying to make sense of them since I wasn't

Am I Ready?

talking to anyone about what had happened.

I didn't check my e-mails. I didn't even watch my favorite TV show, *The Simpsons*. Mom would say, "Your show is on. You're not going to watch it? You're not going to check your e-mail? You've changed since you came back." I felt like telling my mother everything, but I couldn't, not yet. I needed to sort things out first.

Five days later, I decided to see Chris. My plan was to act like a real b-tch, so he'd leave me alone. I didn't want to deal with the constant reminder of that night.

But when I saw Chris, I couldn't even look him in the eyes. We walked on the boardwalk and I was quiet the whole time. Then we went to see his friends. I was still quiet, but I laughed at his friends' jokes. He was sweet and respectful, talking to me calmly and wanting to know things about me. I realized that there was potential for a real relationship, so I decided to see him again.

Seven months later, Chris and I are boyfriend and girlfriend. I'm surprised that the first person I slept with became my guy. I always thought that it would be the other way around: He'd be my guy first and then later we'd be passionate together.

I was so focused on the fact that I'd had sex, I was blind to the clues that he actually liked me.

Our relationship is not simple, though. We've broken up and gotten back together several times. My feelings have changed many times, very fast, from August till now. I hated him, liked him, was annoyed by him, bothered by him, loved him, hated him and loved him. He says that my fluctuating attitude is what bothers him the most about me. I wonder if things would have gone smoother if we'd waited to have sex.

Now that I'm in a relationship, I have a better sense of why I was afraid of relationships before—the emotions can be overwhelming. When I love Chris, he's the best person in the world. But when I feel neglected because he has things to do, I hate him.

When I have things to do, I think he feels bad too, because he'll say something stupid like, "I think this is a sign." I hate that, because he makes it sound like neither of us is committed to the relationship.

But we're working on all that. This relationship is work, but I also think you have to work hard for some of the best things in life, like good grades. I've had sex with Chris since the first time. I enjoy it more now because I have this feeling of love inside me, rather than confused feelings for someone I just met.

The author was 17 when she wrote this story. She graduated from high school and enrolled in college and the U.S. Army.

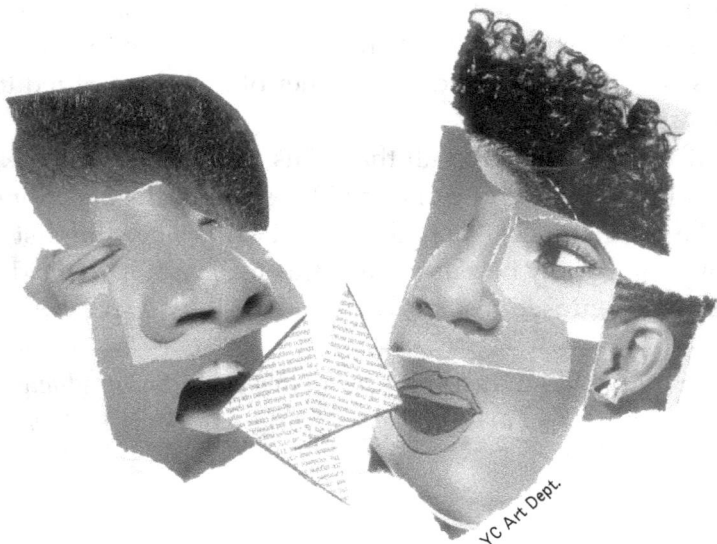

YC Art Dept.

Can We Talk About Sex With Our Parents?

By Anonymous

I was sitting in my room, listening to the music flow through my speakers, when the ringing of the phone interrupted my mood. My mom walked in and asked if I knew that my 15-year-old sister had a boyfriend. She had her phone in her hand, and the intensity in her eyes scared me.

My sister wasn't allowed to have a boyfriend, but I knew she did have one. I was only 12 but she'd trusted me with the secret that she was dating a 19-year-old guy. So I lied and told my mother I didn't know about him.

My mother slammed my door and her anger shook my entire room. She waited for my sister to get out of the shower, still holding her phone tight enough to almost break it. My sister stepped out of the bathroom unaware of the wrath she was about to face.

It was quiet for a few moments but the rage inside my mother was boiling. Finally she couldn't hold on any longer. Her sharp words came out like fire as she yelled at my sister for having sex at such a young age. There was a brief silence, so I walked out into the living room. But as I stepped into the war zone, my mother started shouting again. My sister just kept saying "sorry" over and over.

"I should call the cops to get him arrested since he's too old for you!" my mother yelled. "You're a minor and what he did to you is considered rape. I should put him away for that, so you can never see him again."

Later that day, my mother told me that my sister might be pregnant. My sister had told her friend, and her friend's mother had overheard the conversation and called my mother. After the big fight, my mother grounded my sister and restricted her phone privileges. She didn't forgive my sister for a long time, but she never brought up the issue of my sister having sex again.

Thankfully my sister wasn't pregnant. And after that scare, she didn't have unprotected sex anymore. She told me that she knew what she'd done was wrong and she didn't want to disappoint my mother again.

That look of disappointment in my mother's eyes has kept me from having sex. I just can't hurt her that way. But

My mother's sharp words came out like fire as she yelled at my sister for having sex at such a young age.

witnessing my sister getting yelled at for having sex made me wonder: What's the best way to tell your parents you're sexually active? Should you tell them at all?

On TV shows, I've seen the girl sit her parents down to tell them how much she appreciates all they've done for her. Then she drops the bomb about having sex. At first the parents are shocked, but the boy comes to meet the father and states that his intentions are good. The father approves the match and the boy and girl get married.

Those programs never show the harsh stuff like parents taking their pregnant daughters to the abortion clinic or buying them the morning-after pill. They sugarcoat it so that everyone takes responsibility for their actions and everyone's lives turn out fine.

But that's not real life. My friends who are already having sex tell me they refuse to tell their parents. They say their parents would go mental and probably lock them away for life. After what went down in my house, I wouldn't be surprised.

I wanted to know if and how I should tell my mother when I do become sexually active, so I decided to find out what other teens do. I started my quest at my high school. My classmates talk about sex all the time, so I knew they'd have opinions about it. My former English teacher and I planned a lesson based on my questions.

I wondered how my classmates knew when they were ready to have sex. Most said they got a feeling inside telling them they were ready. "There's no right age to have sex," said Charles, 17.

"As long as you have protection, then why not?" said Isha, 16. "When you're emotionally responsible and can handle the baggage of sex, then it's OK."

Their answers shocked me. I wouldn't want my 14-year-old cousin having sex because she thinks she can handle the emotional baggage. I don't think she's mature enough to handle the pressure that comes along with having sex.

Most students said they hadn't told their parents they were sexually active. Some said it was because they didn't know how to say it, but others said they were scared about how their parents would react. "I wouldn't tell my parents because I know them. My father would try to find out who he is, where he goes to school, and what he looks like," said Karida, 16.

Not everyone agreed with Karida. Dan, 16, said he'd tell his parents if they asked him about it. "Sex would be safer if you told your parents," he said. "Your parents could teach you things [like how to be safe]. And if you don't tell your parents, you could get busted."

I'd never thought that telling your parents that you're having sex might be safer, but he had a point. Some of my classmates thought that teens with strict parents were more likely to have sex. "If your parents are strict, you want to try whatever they don't want you to do," said Talula, 17. "If you have parents who let you do what you want, there's no fun in that."

Some of my classmates thought that teens with strict parents were more likely to have sex.

I don't think that's always true. My mother is strict but I haven't felt the need to go out and have sex.

Even though I knew my mom's take on sex—no sex until college—I wanted to know how I should tell her if I did decide to have sex. I decided to ask her, but I knew that I'd be too grossed out to ask her about sex in person. And having to hear her say the word "sex" would disturb me. So I wrote down several questions and asked her to answer them honestly.

I didn't even read her answers until I was out of the house. I imagined my mother laughing while writing her answers. I read the sarcasm in every word. I'd asked what she'd do if I was pregnant or had a sexually transmitted disease. She'd simply written, "I'll kill you."

I needed her to clarify why, so I overcame my fear and asked her in person when I got home that night. "I raised you not to have sex," she said. "If you were to come home with something that was the result of sex, it means you weren't listening. That makes me look like a bad parent."

Right there, I concluded that what she worried about was how people saw her. I saw her in a different light, because it sounded like all she cared about was how we made her look.

Still, the results of my research made me wonder. Everyone's parents say not to have sex, but many teens do anyway.

Am I Ready?

Why don't I? Maybe it's because my mom doesn't teach me values only by yelling at me. She also validates me at home, telling me that I'm beautiful and special, and that she loves me.

She and other family members surround me with love and support so I don't feel the need to have sex with a person who tells me those things. If more parents did that, maybe their kids wouldn't drop their pants every time someone said they looked good.

Several students said they wanted to tell their parents they were sexually active, but they thought their parents wouldn't understand. But their answers made me wonder. If they're scared about what their parents are going to do, maybe they shouldn't have sex until they leave home.

For me, I think the best way to tell my mother would be when I'm in a sexual relationship with someone I truly care about, but I'll figure that out when the time comes. I don't think I'll start having sex until I move out of my house to go to college. For now, my focus is on school, not sex.

The writer was in high school when she wrote this story.

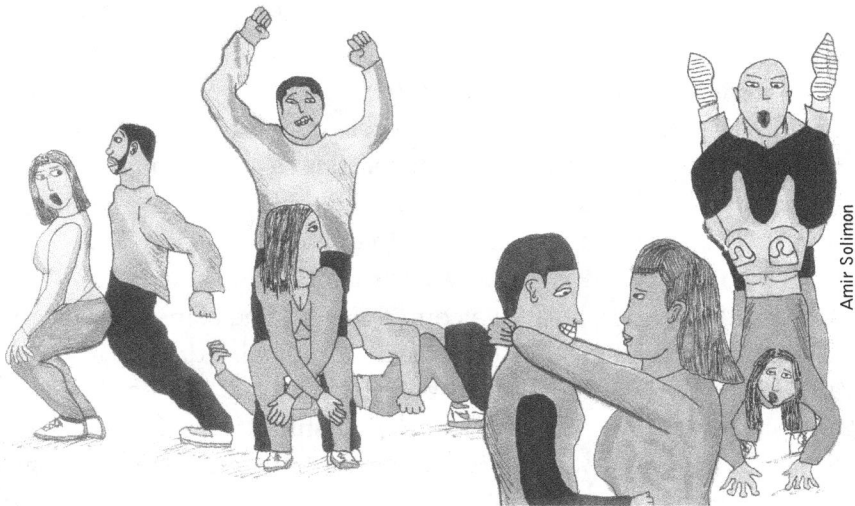

Amir Solimon

Dirty Dancing

By Janill Briones

At its best, dancing's like floating for me. The music possesses me and I can't help but move to the beat. It's a happy feeling, and it's even nicer when I have a dancing partner—one who can dance at least a foot away, or get close without trying anything funny.

Unfortunately, there wasn't any dancing like that at my school's Valentine's Day dance this past February.

I wasn't too excited about the dance when I heard about it. The friends I usually hang out with weren't going, and I didn't want to go all by myself. A ticket cost five bucks, and besides, I figured they'd be playing rap and hip-hop and reggae and none of the type of music that I like to dance to, like salsa and merengue. Why bother to go?

But my friend Jermaine was going and he convinced me to go. "I'll tell you what," he said. "If you don't have fun, I'll personally refund your money."

"All right, I'll go," I said, "but seriously, I want my money back if I don't have fun."

I went home to get ready. My friend from junior high school, Yachira, called and became very excited when I told her that I needed to get ready for the dance. "Have you thought about what you're going to wear?" she asked. "How are you going to do your hair? How are you going to do your makeup?"

The only makeup I usually wear is lip gloss. Yachira asked if she could help out, and I welcomed her to. She came over to my house and helped me pick out an outfit: red shirt, dark blue jeans, and black boots. Then she clipped my hair and curled it down, and shimmered me up with something shiny from the Gap.

Even though it was completely different from the way I usually dress for school, I felt really nice—pretty, if I may say so myself. I began to feel a bit better about going to the dance.

When I arrived at school at 6:15, everyone was at the far end of the gym, away from the dance floor. I took off my coat, spotted my friends and walked toward them. I liked their reaction to the way I was dressed (their mouths dropped), but I was kind of disappointed to see that I was the only one who'd dressed up.

Some people were dancing not too far away from everyone else, but it was hard to tell since everyone was bunched up against the wall. Then I realized that the people on the wall were dancing—just not the way that I dance.

The girls had their backs against the guys' fronts, pushing themselves together and making weird faces. I'd seen people dance like that at my junior high prom and too many times in music videos, but I was still shocked that their dancing was so suggestive. "If that's how everyone's dancing," I thought, "count me out."

Then, my friends tried to make me do it. "Are you out of your mind?" I yelled out over the loud music. "I do not dance like that."

"It's easy, though," my friend said. "Just do it like this." She demonstrated on our friend Anthony (not his real name). It was like Anthony was a car and she was using her butt to clean him, in a circular motion.

Yeah, it seemed simple enough, but I still didn't like the idea of rubbing myself on a guy's—front. I asked my friends what they thought about dancing like that, and they said that it was just fun for them. It was as if it were no big deal to display sexual activity.

It was like Anthony was a car and she was using her butt to clean him.

I think it's OK to show off that you like someone, and maybe even flirt and kiss in public, but that's about it. Everything else should be done in private, not where everyone else can see it. That kind of stuff is supposed to be intimate.

Without warning, my friends pushed me up against Anthony and encouraged me to "dance." I didn't last two seconds before I had to step away. I just couldn't do it. It was gross.

I went over to Jermaine to complain about his guarantee on my having fun. "That isn't dancing," I said. "That's just people smooshing themselves together and rolling around—coincidentally with music in the background. I should have brought my book." He laughed.

Over the evening, the dancing became more outrageous. I stood there intrigued and appalled at the same time. Some of the girls were on the floor, with the guy on top of them. Others weren't even touching ground as they hung on to their dancing partner like a monkey clinging to its owner. One girl was upside-down, on her hands, while a guy held her legs—wide open—while he pushed on her. "That's not dancing," I kept telling myself. "That's sex with clothes on."

I hardly danced, and when I did, it was either by myself or with my female friends. I danced (my way) with just two guys, Anthony and Jermaine. The rest of the guys I knew wouldn't dance with me if I didn't push myself all up on them.

Anthony preferred to dance with "easier-going" girls. Only Jermaine seemed to not mind. (Maybe it was the guilt of convincing me to go.) But when I was dancing with him, a girl swooped in and pushed her back up on him, stealing my dancing partner.

It was such a relief when I got home. It felt nice to get away. The horror of what I had just experienced still loomed. I thought maybe those girls felt so comfortable engaging in public sexual display because they had already had sex. "Are they so proud of being sexually active that they have to show it off to everyone?" I wondered.

I'd heard girls at my school talk about losing their virginity as if it were no big deal. It made me feel awkward, because that's not how I see it. But I know that we also see public displays of sex all the time in movies and TV shows, and especially music videos. We teens are being deluded into believing that life is all about sex. I can't help but wonder why we would want to grow up so quickly.

"That's not dancing," I said. "That's sex with clothes on."

Jermaine gave me my $5 back when we got to school the next day, but I know he won't always be there to refund my money. Now I worry that the prom will be just like the Valentine's Day dance, or worse. At least the friends I usually hang out with will be there, so maybe I'll feel more comfortable.

I'm not giving in to what everyone else is doing, though. And if no one wants to dance with me because I won't dance dirty, then there is nothing wrong with floating alone.

Janill was 15 when she wrote this story. She later graduated from college with a degree in psychology.

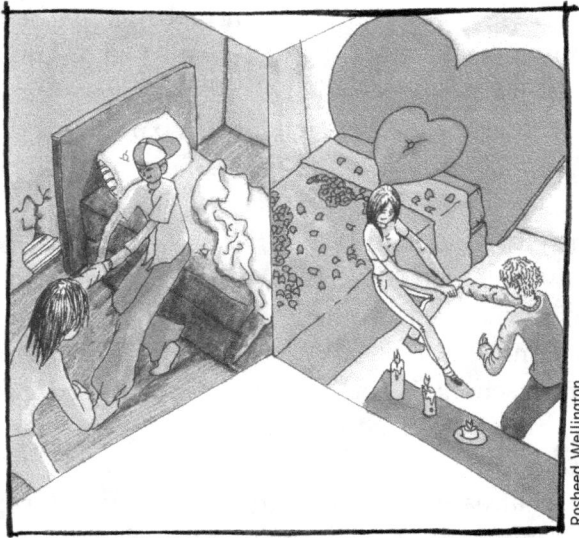

Rosheed Wellington

It Takes Love to Make Love

By Anonymous

Carlos was South American but looked European—tall and light-skinned with short black hair. It was obvious other girls liked him because of the shameless flirting they directed toward him. But I didn't like him or flirt with him. He was arrogant and constantly bragged about his magnificent country, Chile.

"My country is better than yours, there is no discussion," he'd start.

"Are you talking to me?" I'd reply.

"Yeah! You're Mexican, right?"

"Yes, so what?"

"Mexican girls are too dark, not like Chilean girls," he'd say with a sly smile.

"I don't care. I like it there. At least in Mexico I didn't have to meet people like you," I'd say and walk away in disgust.

Am I Ready?

All this was said in Spanish, since we'd only been in New York about two weeks and didn't know a word of English. It was very difficult for me because I was 15 and was living with my mom and brother for the first time, and I barely knew them.

Carlos and I had that kind of argument every day at lunch, sitting at the cafeteria table with the other Spanish-speaking newcomers. His bragging made me furious.

But slowly he grew on me. We were always in the same classes and sat near each other. He started talking to me about his life, his family, and his customs. One day he told me he liked someone from school. I thought it was one of my friends and told him I could help him if he told me who it was. That Friday, he asked me out.

By then I already liked him a lot but I was surprised, so I told him I'd think about it over the weekend. Even though I felt flattered and happy, I didn't know what to think because the day before I'd seen him talking to my friend in the same close way he'd been talking to me.

But I decided to go out with him, and the following Monday after school we had our first kiss. His kiss felt refreshing, like a glass of cold water on a hot summer day. Still, I couldn't help but think of my first kiss ever, back in Mexico when I was 13.

Angel had short, curly black hair, dark eyes, and a caramel complexion that matched his sweetness. He was 19, and Dad didn't want me to have a boyfriend, let alone someone that much older than me. "A boy that old only wants sex from you!" he said.

But I'd never been so happy. Angel was always there for me, writing poems, quoting big poets, thinking of a life with me. He took every single step as slow as I wanted him to. It was a week and a half before we had our first kiss, and only because I wanted to. He always said I was the most important thing in his life and that he'd never hurt me if he could avoid it. I never doubted him.

The sex theme came up a few times, usually when I brought it up because I was concerned that he might have sex with someone else. Angel told me he wasn't a virgin but that he would wait until I was ready.

When we kissed, I felt an incredible desire that I believed couldn't be bad. But I was too scared. My religion prohibits sex before marriage. My family disapproved of it and I wasn't ready to break the rules just yet. But we didn't need sex for our relationship to grow strong, though my father grew madder about it, and even threatened Angel's life.

Eventually my father won his fight by taking me to another city and restricting my every step. Since I didn't have a phone, Angel and I slowly fell out of touch. Angel would try to see me every weekend, but we could only see each other through the window. My father started telling me stories of how he'd seen Angel with other girls. Eventually I believed Dad and broke up with Angel.

Instead of making us feel closer, having sex pushed us further apart.

But now those days of my first love were over. I felt good thinking that this new kiss was as meaningful for Carlos as it was for me.

Our relationship was happy at first. Then, a month into it, Carlos asked me, "Don't you think we should have sex?" I didn't know how I felt about having sex with him. Plus, I was a virgin and I didn't know if I wanted to stop being one. He said it was all going to be OK, but I told him I wasn't ready. I didn't think he was worth losing my virginity to. I wasn't sure I trusted him.

Over the next two months we talked about it on the phone almost every day. He'd start by telling me he loved me and somehow he'd bring up the subject out of nowhere. Sometimes I'd try to ignore it, but other times I'd respond.

"I don't think we're ready to do it now," I'd say.

Am I Ready?

"Why not? If not now, when?" he'd ask.

That was our main discussion, in person and by phone. He had me thinking about it all day and the pressure grew stronger all the time. I felt like a bug caught in a spider's web.

Finally, two months later, I gave in. I couldn't take it anymore. I wanted to believe all his sweet talk was true. I told myself that if we did it, it was going to be done with love and that he'd be sweet. But his constant pressuring had made me start to like him less, and I worried that he only wanted to use me.

I told him that I was going to do it with him, but I also expressed my fear. "I don't want it to hurt. They say it hurts—a lot," I said. And, "You'll probably want to leave me after we do it." He never really said anything about those comments. That's when I felt that he was a fake.

So how could I do it? Trust me, I've asked myself that same question several times and I still don't know. But everything happened so fast, so nightmare-like, that I didn't even realize what was going on.

When it started happening, I asked myself so many questions. "Am I doing the right thing? Is Mom going to be mad at me? Is this the right person? Am I thinking about Angel?"

I answered myself in two seconds. "Yes! Maybe. It has to be. No way—that was a long time ago!" But the answers didn't really matter, because while I was thinking all that, he was taking my pants off.

One moment we were kissing and the next, my pants were down. He'd said he was a virgin, but he certainly didn't act like I thought one would. He was kind of rough and fast and seemed secure about what was he was doing.

The next thing I knew, it was over. I was in his living room sitting on his sofa. Something hurt, and I looked down to where blood was coming out and tears started to fall from my eyes.

"What's wrong?" he asked.

"I don't know!" I said. "Why did we do this?"

"Because we love each other."

I didn't think so. I hated him then and felt like all he said was lies. We'd used a condom, but that didn't make me feel any better. It was done and couldn't be undone or erased no matter how much I wanted to erase it. It just didn't feel right. There was a lack of something—emotion, love, maybe passion.

Instead of making us feel closer, having sex pushed us further apart. I didn't tell Carlos that I didn't feel anything good physically or emotionally. I didn't tell him how when I went home that day, I took the longest bath I've ever taken, hoping to wash away the day. I didn't tell him that I felt he was a liar.

Sex with Carlos was all I'd feared it would be: cold, unsentimental, indifferent.

I think I was trying to spare the feelings I thought he had. And I hoped it would be better the next time. But when we did it at his house again a few weeks later, I still didn't feel a thing. Everything was like the first time, just faster.

*E*ven so, I kept on dating Carlos. By the second year of our relationship I was certain that making love was a lie, a cruel myth. Sex with Carlos was all I'd feared it would be: cold, unsentimental, indifferent. Every time we did it, I felt like running away. I was impressed that he could be so cold when he was so sweet at times. And I didn't understand why I kept doing it. I always felt trapped during and after sex.

Somehow it all kept going, the sex and our relationship, even though I didn't enjoy the sex and our relationship was only one problem after another, mostly over rumors that he was with another girl or I was with another boy. We broke up often, but then he'd convince me that our love was worth it, or I would convince him.

I guess I stayed because I didn't want to go from man to man.

I was afraid that no one would ever respect me again, and that he was the only one who would want me, since I was no longer a virgin.

Throughout all this time I never told anyone what was going on. I had told my mom that I was no longer a virgin and she wasn't mad. But I never told her how horrible sex was with Carlos. Then, nearly three years into my relationship with Carlos, my father decided to take my brother and me to Mexico for the summer.

Soon after we arrived in Mexico, I went to stay with my cousin Margaret. I learned that she and Angel were still in touch, so Angel knew I was going to be at her house for almost three weeks. When she told me he was coming to see me, I got very excited.

That night I broke up with Carlos by phone and didn't call him for the rest of the summer. It was easier to break up with him from so far away. I felt free knowing I wouldn't see him for a long time and that helped me detach myself from him.

The next day Angel came over, and I felt like my 14-year-old self again—happy, trusting, nervous, naïve, excited—the person I missed being. Angel always had that effect on me.

Three days later he kissed me. I told him I had broken up with my boyfriend very recently. Angel just said that he wasn't going to make me do anything that I didn't want to do.

Then I decided that I wanted to see if he could make love to me. I thought maybe I'd like it since we knew each other so well and I still felt a connection with him. I didn't tell him, but the next time we saw each other I kissed him and he knew. He always had a way of knowing what I wanted to say without me saying it.

After our first official date, and I mean the first one ever, we decided to do it. Well, I decided to do it. He kissed me and I knew what he was asking me without words. We just looked at each other and I said, "Yes, let's go!" and he took me to his house.

Earlier that afternoon, we had talked about something he noticed when I kissed him. He said it was different because I didn't seem as innocent as I used to be.

He told me he thought I wasn't a virgin and I said he was right. He didn't mind that I wasn't a virgin, though. He said, "Well, I can't ask you to be a nun when I haven't been a saint."

It was almost 1 a.m. when we reached his house that night. He told me to stay outside for a moment. He ran in, came back out with a piece of fabric and wrapped it around my eyes so I couldn't see. He led me to his room and when I took off the

That night I discovered that making love is not a myth, that sexuality can be enjoyed.

blindfold, there was my dream come true: rose petals on the bed and candles all over. He told me he wanted me to remember that night forever.

Not only do I remember that night like it was yesterday, I'm also very grateful, because that night I discovered that making love is not a myth, that sexuality can be enjoyed. He did everything I thought he was supposed to do, demonstrated interest in my enjoyment and was as sweet with me as could be—the total opposite of Carlos.

When I had sex the first time with Carlos, our relationship changed. The time that we'd once spent alone talking was replaced by time alone having sex. But with Angel, we grew closer after we had sex. We talked more and were relaxed and content together. And as I grew more confident with my sexuality, I also grew more confident of myself and of my uniqueness.

I think that the main reason I was with Carlos is that I had a poor opinion of myself. I felt like I had to please him so he'd stay with me, and I didn't think pleasing myself mattered. I didn't love myself enough, so I needed somebody who would promise to love me, no matter what the cost. Gradually, I gave him total control over my feelings and my life.

But thanks to Angel, I learned that demanding and knowing what you want from the person you are having a relationship with is not a crime. It's actually very healthy and natural to want something and ask for it, as long as you give something in return.

From now on I know I need to be my own person, my own confidence booster, and speak my mind whenever I feel uncomfortable. I've decided that whoever wants to be with me in the future needs to want me for what I am and also for what I am not. If the relationship is going wrong, I'll no longer stay quiet and take it. And if I don't want to have sex, I won't have sex, period.

The author was 18 when she wrote this story.

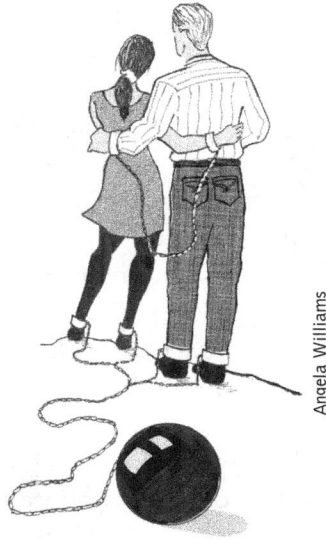

Angela Williams

Single, Happy, and Free

By Irma Johnson

Every teenager should date. If you don't date, there's something wrong with you. If you don't have a boyfriend or girlfriend—go get one! That's the message that television, magazines, and our friends give us.

Open any teen magazine and you'll find at least one article on how to get or keep a boyfriend. Look at the advertisements and you'll learn what perfume to buy to attract a guy. Watch any sitcom and you'll see so-called teenagers going on dates or struggling to attract the opposite sex. Talk to a group of teenage boys hanging out and you'll hear exaggerated accounts of their conquests. It sometimes seems that everyone over 12 is dating. So I interviewed some teenagers in New York City to find out for myself.

The media make it seem like "we're all boy-crazy or girl-crazy and have nothing better to do," says Sharmila Harrinarine, 16. But not everyone is dating—not even close. Sharmila doesn't date because her parents don't think she's old enough. She doesn't mind that much because she doesn't like the guys she meets anyway. "They have too much of an ego, they're fake," she says.

Tonya Bobo, 16, says that her parents won't let her date because they think boys only want sex. Tonya thinks they're probably right. Other teenagers don't date because they haven't found the right person. "I don't meet anyone interesting who asks me out," says Bunni Tan, 15. "The ones who ask me out aren't interesting and the ones who are interesting don't ask me out."

Felix Nicelescu, 16, says that a lot of the girls he meets are "unreal, they're posers," so he has no interest in going out with them. A lot of teenagers who have dated found that it wasn't as great as they thought it would be. Elsie Hsieh, 16, had what some people might consider the perfect boyfriend. He would buy her flowers, take her out to lunch, and give her presents.

But Elsie quickly got sick of doing "everything people expected us to do." She has decided that she's "not going out with a guy again unless we're good friends first.... I won't date for the hell of it! What's the point? Just to say I have a boyfriend?"

Yudi Persaud, 15, had a girlfriend but it didn't work out. "She brought my level of confidence down so I became more timid in front of girls," Yudi says. Now Yudi's not dating and has girls as friends instead. Felix admits that one reason he doesn't date is that he's scared of rejection.

Friends and the media can make teenagers who don't date feel that there is something wrong with them. This can be especially true for boys. According to Wendy Yalowitz, clinical supervisor at the Youth Counseling League in Manhattan, "Boys are under an extreme amount of pressure to take the initiative." Yudi agrees. "Every guy has to have a story about some 'event,'" he says.

Even teens who are comfortable with not dating feel they are missing out on some things. "Girls who date have someone to walk the halls with, to confide in, to be there," Sharmila says. Tonya says she sometimes wishes she knew "how it feels to be in love and all that mushy stuff. Sometimes I feel a little sad, lonely." Yudi says he too would like to have "someone to be intimate with." Without a girlfriend, he gets "bored once in a while, sometimes lonesome."

But teenagers who aren't dating are not necessarily unhappy. Most spend lots of time hanging out with friends, studying, or working. "I'm not missing enjoying myself," says Matthew Keith, 17. "I have friends to go out with. I go out more now than when I did date. I'm having fun." Many teens agree with Bunni Tan, whose attitude towards dating is "if it happens, fine. If it doesn't, I'm not going to kill myself over it."

Elsie Hsieh says, "I see a lot of advantages with not dating.... I see friends who get so tied up. I don't think I can handle the emotional ties." Sharmila agrees. "My friends [who date] seem more depressed, like they have more on their minds...always worried about something," she says.

So if you're not dating, relax! You're not abnormal. There's nothing wrong with you. "People are ready [to date] at different stages of their teenage years," said Yalowitz. "People have to go at their own pace." In the long run, not dating as a teenager may even make you a stronger, more independent person. As Matthew Keith says, "You've got to be mature to feel good about yourself and not date."

Irma was 16 when she wrote this story. She later graduated from college and worked for a nonprofit youth program and a grantmaker.

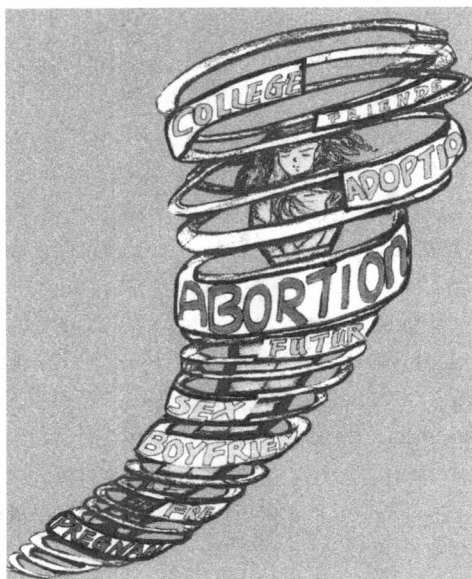

Yan Hua-Deng

The Right Choice—for Now

By Anonymous

When I was 17 years old and two weeks away from being done with 10th grade, my old boyfriend called me. I say "old" and not "ex" because I always seemed to get back with him when he came back into the city on vacations from college.

Our relationship started when I was in 9th grade and he was a senior. It started out slow. For a long time, we just talked and walked around. But, by the end of the school year, the relationship had become very sexual. I didn't have a big problem with this. He was not my first; I had had sex before. And I always wanted to see him.

When he called to say he was home from college, the topic of seeing each other came up. I said, "Sure. How 'bout this week?" I had half days at school all week. He picked me up in his car, and we drove toward his house.

I knew that sex was on both of our minds but I didn't want to talk about it. I guess I felt embarrassed after not seeing him for a while. In the car, we joked around and held hands but didn't say anything about sex. We talked about school and what we were doing with our lives.

When we got to his house, it all seemed nice and calm at first. We were just watching TV and laughing about the stupid topics that the talk shows were about.

After an hour of flipping back and forth between shows, I felt the feeling of sex come over my body. It was like an urge that pushed me forward. I felt a little scared, but I also wanted to do this. We kissed a little and then we went to it.

While it was happening, I was thinking two things at once. One thing was, "This is the right thing to do." The other was, "What the heck am I doing?" I was thinking that maybe this wasn't such a good thing for me because I hadn't seen him in a while. I guess the "this is right" took over because I didn't stop.

Afterwards, we hung around his house for a while and then he drove me back home. I wanted to see him again but neither of us called the other. I'm not exactly sure why.

About two weeks later, I started to feel strange. My body was aching all the time, and going up and down stairs was harder than usual. I just pushed the thought of being pregnant out of my mind. I thought a little bit about it but didn't want it to be real. I thought, "How could that happen?"

After I started getting sick every morning, my mom asked me if I thought I was pregnant. I said, "Maybe." Then I said, "Yes."

My mom was very helpful about it. She didn't get all mad at me. I was the one who was the most upset. I started to cry. I was so scared of what might happen.

We went to the doctor and I found out that I was seven weeks pregnant. The doctor asked me what I wanted to do. I told her that I would think about it and call her to let her know. A lot of things were going through my mind. I was in shock about being pregnant. I was afraid of having an operation. But I knew that it was best for me to have an abortion.

I knew that I wasn't ready to be a mother to a child. I love children, but the thought of being a single mother was scary. I knew that my mother would help me as much as she could, but she has a job and can't take care of a baby all day long. I would also have to go to school in the last months of my pregnancy and that would be horrible.

I knew that I wasn't ready to be a mother.

I knew that this would be the gossip for years to come. My school is so small that everyone knows everybody else. I knew I would be teased and tortured and I didn't want that at all. Besides, I had dreams of going to college. Having a baby would have made me have to rethink my future.

And I wouldn't have the kind of support that a father can give: I didn't even tell my old boyfriend I was pregnant. I was scared about what he might say. I thought that he would just deny that anything had happened and say that it wasn't him. I didn't think I would be able to deal with that.

It was a very short time before I told my doctor that I wanted to have an abortion. The thought of getting sick, of having a baby, and of being pregnant at school made the choice clear. I talked about it with my best friends. At first they were mostly shocked, but then they wanted to talk about it and try and help me. Even after making the decision, I was still really crazed and nervous. My friends made me calm down a lot.

The day of the abortion, I woke up scared. I have never liked pain or operations. I didn't want to go at first, but my mom told me that I had made the right decision for myself. I was still nervous when I got to the hospital but I went into the room and sat down and waited for the doctor.

My doctor was very nice to me and told me what she was going to do before she started. She gave me a lot of painkillers but the procedure still hurt. I was mostly awake the whole time. I wasn't really thinking about anything during it.

Afterward, they put me in a wheelchair and brought me into a room that was full of people who were recovering from different operations. The nurse asked me if I wanted anything and I told her I was thirsty. When she came back, I asked her if I could go see my mom. I didn't want to stay in that room. It was too scary. There were too many other people around. I just wanted to see my mom and go home. I was really tired. When I got home, I slept for a long time.

More than a year has passed since then. I still think about the abortion a lot. Sometimes I wish I'd had the baby.

I finally talked to my old boyfriend again and told him that he had gotten me pregnant. His reaction was just the opposite of what I thought. He said that he would have helped me with the baby or at least would have liked to be with me when I had the abortion. When I found that out, I felt a little bad that I didn't tell him. But, at the time, I was really mad at him for doing this to me. I didn't think about his feelings that much.

Because of the pregnancy, I'm much more careful about sex and protection now.

I still think that it was best for me to finish school before having a baby, but I feel sad that I had to have an abortion to make that possible. If I was out of high school, I think I would have had the baby. But school was much too important to me at the time. Not to mention giving up all my free time and not being able to hang out with my friends whenever I wanted.

Because of the pregnancy, I'm much more careful about sex and protection now. I feel like I have to be extremely careful and make sure everything is right before sex. After I had the abortion, I started taking the Pill even though I don't really want to have sex that much anymore. When I do want to, I will make sure I feel safe and happy with the person I'm with.

I know that I really want to have a baby when I meet the right man and I feel it's the right time for me. But it's not that time yet.

The writer was 18 when she wrote this story.

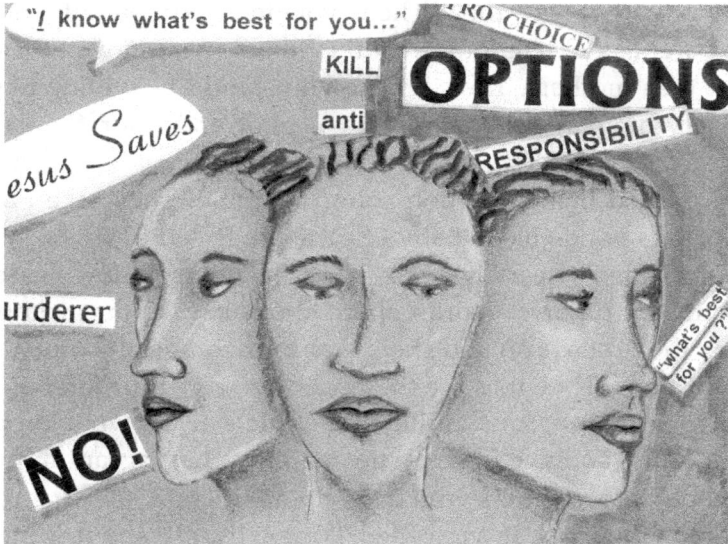

"I know what's best for you..."

KILL **OPTIONS**

PRO CHOICE

anti

esus Saves

RESPONSIBILITY

urderer

"what's best for you?"

NO!

Melanie Leong

Scare Tactics

By Anonymous

Last year, I planned to write an article about both sides of the abortion debate. I started off at a pro-life place called Expectant Mother Care (EMC) in New York City. I wanted to know more about their beliefs and what they do.

Before I went I was unsure about what abortion was or how I felt about it. I did not know what all the fuss was about. EMC advertises itself as being against abortion, so I spoke to a counselor there. What I found out was a little more than I could handle.

They believe abortion is wrong, so they try to scare teens into having their babies and they make it seem like it is easy to take care of a child. First they tell you the ways that you can get support during and after pregnancy. They tell you they'll give you a year's supply of baby products. Then they encourage you to switch schools to a high school for teen mothers.

Finally, they say they'll help you tell your parents, and if your parents kick you out, then they'll help you move to a shelter for teen mothers. They act like you should be willing to give up everything in your life—your school and your family—to become a teen mother.

They also make abortion sound horrible. They take out an object that sounds like a baby's heartbeat. If you have the slightest thing called a heart, it makes you want to break down in tears. They make up horror stories about abortion (like that you'll die during the procedure) and show you a videotape of women having abortions. They told me these women were murderers.

They also gave me a million pamphlets about what happens to the fetus, about females who regretted having an abortion, and about teen mothers who had kept their child. One pamphlet struck me the most. It was called "Tragic Diary" and it went like this:

> *October 5: Today my life began. My parents do not know it yet. I am small as the pollen of a flower, but it is I already. I will be a girl. I will have blonde hair and blue eyes. Nearly everything is settled already, even that I shall love flowers.*

> *December 24: I am almost able to see, though it is night around me. When mother brings me into the world, it will be full of sunshine and overflowing with flowers. I have never seen a flower, you know. But more than anything, I want to see my mother. How do you look, Mom?*

> *December 28: Today my mother killed me.*

I couldn't believe what I was reading. I felt like this must be how the baby feels. I started to cry. I felt like I could not live if I had been this baby's mother, and I wondered how a woman could live with herself after having an abortion.

After I left, I was in shock. I felt sick. But I was also confused.

The EMC counselor acted like abortion is the worst thing in the world, but I still wanted to know the other side of the story. If it's so bad, then why is it legal? So I decided to educate myself by reading books and talking to friends and family about what they think. But that didn't help. Everyone was so against it that they couldn't even talk about it. By then I was pretty sure it was wrong. Still, I didn't think I had to make up my mind because I wasn't even having sex yet.

But I guess things happen. A few months later, I was raped. Because I had been there before, I went to EMC to have the pregnancy test. It was positive. When the counselor told me I was pregnant, he talked to me about keeping the baby. He told me I could either stay home or, if my parents threw me out, go to a group home.

He had some decent advice—when I told him that I wanted to go to a group home, he said it would be better for me to stay at home, and that I should tell my parents right away. He said that without my parents, I would feel like I had no support. But he was also clearly opposed to me having an abortion.

After that, I was so confused, but eventually I told my parents. At the time, I wanted to keep the baby. But when I told them, they forced me to have an abortion.

I was against it with full force. Not me, I could not, I would not. I cried every night. I wanted to be a mother, although I knew I was not ready to be one. I kept thinking about what they told me at EMC the first time I went: that I would die during the procedure and that, if I lived, I would be labeled a murderer.

The counselor had some decent advice, but he was also clearly opposed to me having an abortion.

When I went to the abortion clinic with my parents, I was shaking. In the recovery room, I spoke to other girls. They had so many stories about why they were there. Many said they had children already and they could not handle having another, and others said they didn't want any kids yet.

I felt a bit strange. They acted like an abortion was a common thing to do and so was sex. I thought to myself, "These girls need to use some type of contraceptive if they want to have sex." I felt angry at them.

Afterwards I was fine, physically, but I regretted having the abortion. I had seen the sonogram, and saw the baby inside, and I got so attached. I did feel relieved not to have to be a mother. But I also felt shocked and sad: I felt like I had killed my child. It was only when I started school again, and realized how much I would have had to change if I had kept my baby, that I was glad I didn't.

After that, I knew I never wanted to have another abortion again. So even though I'm not having sex, I made an appointment at Planned Parenthood, where teenagers can get birth control for free, so I could go on the Pill and never get pregnant again.

When I went, I wished I had gone to Planned Parenthood in the first place. It's better to learn the facts about abortion and get counseling that helps you decide what you want for yourself than to get scared at an anti-abortion place like EMC.

Almost a year later, I went back to EMC to talk to the counselor I had first met. This time, I saw two black girls in the waiting room. They were my age. When I saw them, I felt outraged, because I knew the counselor was about to scare them just like she scared me. She would make it sound like it's some kind of fantasy raising a child, even though she has no idea what a 15-year-old is going through or how her life will change.

I thought, "These little girls are faced with such a big decision and all that lady can do is tell them her beliefs, not try to help them make the best decision." I wished I could have rushed those girls out of there and straight to Planned Parenthood, where they offer information and they help you form your own opinion. The counselors are there to help you make a decision, not to get you to do what they think you should do.

After all I've been through, I feel like I am finally sure of what

I believe: that if you are faced with a situation where an abortion might be the best choice for you, then no one should stand in your way.

I don't believe that people can understand why females have an abortion unless they are faced with it themselves. If you think you can know your mind without having to face being pregnant and unprepared, then I think you are just fooling yourself. I should know. I regret having to have an abortion, but it was the best thing for me at the time, and I am sure other girls who have had an abortion would say the same thing.

> *I don't believe that people can understand why females have an abortion unless they are faced with it themselves.*

I don't think people who work in places like the EMC clinic can really understand the girls who walk in the door, and how it's going to change their lives to have a child. They don't care about what's best for the girl's life. It seems to me that it's all about their religion and getting points to enter heaven. Once the girl has her child and they're both struggling—well, that part is not the counselors' problem.

The writer was 17 when she wrote this story.

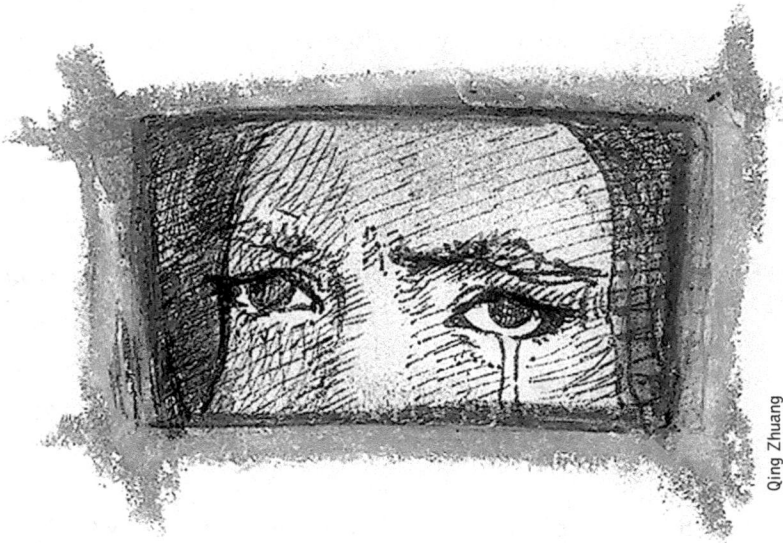
Qing Zhuang

I Paid the Price for Unprotected Sex—Twice

By Anonymous

It all began when I broke my virginity, three years ago. I was 14 years old and just starting puberty. I was new to sex and to all the good and bad things that can happen to a girl. I've learned a lot since then, but I learned it the hard way.

This guy I knew back then kept on talking about sex and all these things that we could try. So, I kind of fell into something that I thought was going to be good for me without really thinking about where it might lead. I could say that it was all his fault because he kept on filling my head with all these sexual images when he knew that I was still very young and a virgin. But, on the other hand, the things he said felt really good and I wanted to try them.

For about a year and a half, I had unprotected sex and it didn't occur to me that I could catch something or even get pregnant. I was never really taught a lot about sex and diseases—maybe that's why. I just didn't think that condoms were necessary. My attitude was, if the guy didn't want to use a condom, then he must be clean. I trusted him. I really never asked a guy to use one: The words just wouldn't come out of my mouth.

I thought about telling my ex to get tested, but I was angry at him for giving me this thing.

Then, one day, my mother read my diary. When she found out that I wasn't a virgin anymore, she flipped. She told me that she was disappointed in me, that I should have waited. She was also concerned that I was having unprotected sex, so she hooked me up with the free clinic across the street from where we live.

On my first visit, they did an examination, took blood to run some tests and took urine for a pregnancy test. Then they told my mother, who had come with me, that I was just fine.

After that, I continued having unprotected sex. About six months later, I started to have serious cramping in my abdomen. I didn't pay attention to it for about six or seven months, because my period was very irregular at that time and I thought the cramps were just my period telling me, "I'm on my way, so be prepared." Then the clinic sent me a letter saying that my annual checkup was due, so they made an appointment for me to come in.

On that particular visit, they did a pap smear and tested me for STDs. When the results came back, I got a major scare. They said that I had gotten something called chlamydia, a bacterial infection you can get from having unprotected sex. I almost dropped down and cried.

The nurse at the clinic said that it was curable. She gave me some medication to drink and told me it would take seven days to work and that I shouldn't have sex again until after that.

The nurse also said that my sex partners must be treated too, or they could give it to me again, or to someone else.

A little information about this bacteria. Whoever contracts it can give it to someone else if they have unprotected sex together. And chlamydia may be curable, but it is still very dangerous to a person's reproductive organs. It can prevent a woman from having children in the future, because you can become sterile if the bacteria goes untreated for too long.

After my appointment, I thought about telling my ex to get tested, but I was angry at him for giving me this thing and, even if I did want to tell him, I couldn't, because he was nowhere to be found. I think that he left the state to go away on a trip, and I couldn't call him because I'd lost his phone number.

After the chlamydia cleared up, I went back to having unprotected sex because I thought that my new boyfriend was clean. Besides, in the heat of the moment, I just didn't want to stop to put a condom on.

Chlamydia can prevent a woman from having children in the future.

After a few months had passed, I started to experience the same cramps in my stomach, so I set up another appointment to see the doctor. They did some tests and found out that the chlamydia was back.

I was on my way to realizing that I may never have kids in the future. Over the past three years, I have had numerous partners and I didn't care enough about myself to ever say, "Hey, put a condom on," because I didn't have my head on straight. When I went out with a guy, we never discussed using protection. Because some guys don't feel comfortable using condoms, I just got used to the not-using-a-condom thing.

But unprotected sex can lead to a whole lot of unwanted things. Contracting this disease twice made me very angry at myself and much more scared, because now I realize that if I could get chlamydia twice, I could also have gotten pregnant or gotten AIDS. I know I've got to take sex—and my body—more seriously.

The writer was in high school when she wrote this story.

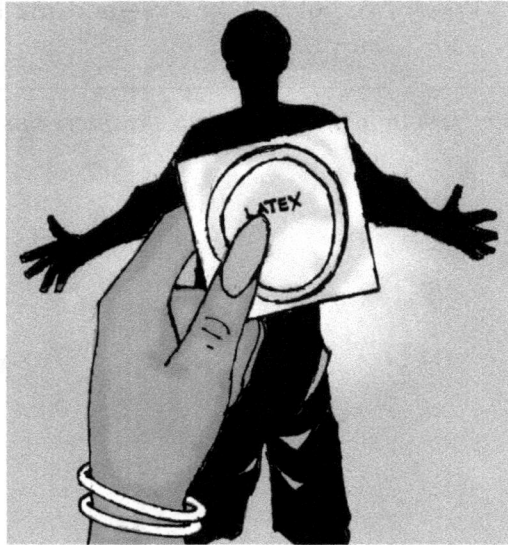

Tangie Bryan

Sexually Transmitted Diseases: Protect Yourself and Your Partner

The last thing you want to do when you're having sex is get a disease, or give one to your partner. Sexually transmitted diseases (STDs; also called sexually transmitted infections or STIs) are very serious, but you can take steps to protect yourself and your partner. Here's what you need to know:

Who gets STDs?

The sad fact is that teens and young adults are most likely to be infected. There are about 19 million new STD infections each year, almost half of them among people ages 15 to 24. A recent study estimated that 1 in every 4 teen girls has been infected with at least one of the four most common STDs (chlamydia, genital herpes, HPV and trichomoniasis).

How do you get an STD?

STDs are primarily spread through sexual contact such as vaginal sex (penis to vagina) anal sex (penis to anus), or oral sex (penis, vagina, or anus to mouth). If you are having sex, you are at risk of getting an STD, regardless of whether you are having sex with women, men, or both.

How can you prevent STDs?

The only completely sure way is to practice abstinence (don't have sex). If you are sexually active, using a barrier method, like a condom every time you have sex, including oral sex, will reduce your risk.

How do you treat an STD?

Trichomoniasis, chlamydia, gonorrhea, and syphilis can be cured with antibiotics. Be careful—after being cured, you can still get re-infected.

Herpes and HIV (the virus that causes AIDS) have no cure—they stay in your body for life. But medication can help reduce the symptoms.

There is also no treatment for HPV, which can cause genital warts and some cancers. But it can be prevented with a new vaccine, which can protect you against the strain of HPV that causes most cases of cervical cancer. Ask your doctor about the vaccine—it's best if you get it before becoming sexually active.

For more information on specific STDs, their symptoms, and how to treat them, check out Planned Parenthood's teen website: plannedparenthood.org/teen-talk.

Who should get tested?

If you've ever had sex, you should get tested for HIV and other STDs. Even if you've had protected sex, you should still get tested periodically, since no method is 100% effective. You can get tested at your doctor's office or at a clinic like Planned Parenthood. Free and low-cost services are available, and you don't need a parent or guardian's permission. They don't have to know about the tests or the results.

For more information, and to find a testing center near you, visit www.hivtest.org, a website run by the Centers for Disease Control and Prevention.

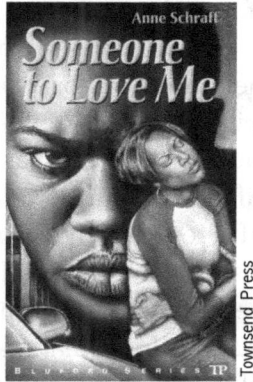

Someone to Love Me

Cindy Gibson tripped over a stack of magazines in the middle of the living room, bumped her knee against the sharp corner of the coffee table, and dropped a can of cat food on the floor.

"Ouch, my leg!" she howled. "This place is a freakin' mess!" Her two cats, Theo and Cleo, scurried beneath the table.

Lorraine, Cindy's mother, came out of her bedroom carrying a small mirror. She peered at her reflection as she walked, carefully examining the lipstick she had just put on. "Stop whinin', baby. Just straighten things up before you leave for school. I'm late for work."

"I'm not going to school today," Cindy declared. She waited to see if her mother would get angry and insist that she go. Cindy was a freshman at Bluford High, and even though it was only October, she had already missed several days of school.

Here's the first chapter from *Someone to Love Me*, by Anne Schraff, a novel about a girl facing difficult situations like the ones you read about in this book. *Someone to Love Me* is one of several books in the Bluford Series™ by Townsend Press.

"You better go to school, baby," her mother said, touching up her eye makeup. "If you drop out at your age, you'll end up like me, in your thirties waitin' tables at some grease pit for next to nothing. This ain't the kinda life you wanna have, girl. Believe me on that. By the way, if Raffie calls, tell him I'm off work at five tonight. Bye, baby." Cindy heard a thud as her mother closed the front door of their small apartment.

Theo, a jet-black cat, crept warily from under the table, followed by Cleo, who was gray and white. Dust and crumbs from under the table stuck delicately to each cat's coat.

Cindy brushed the cats' fur, cleaned up the spilled food, and walked out to the kitchen. Theo and Cleo followed quickly behind her. "Mom doesn't really care if I go to school," Cindy pouted, grabbing a fresh can of cat food. "All she cares about is Raffie and whether or not she's put the right gunk on her face, right, Theo?" The cat blinked and rubbed its furry face against her leg.

Theo and Cleo were Cindy's best friends. She told them everything. They were there for her whenever she was lonely or needed someone to talk to. It was more than she could say for Mom, Cindy thought.

"I ain't goin' anywhere today, Cleo. I'm stayin' right here and watchin' trashy talk shows all day. I don't care what Mom says," Cindy said, spooning chunks of cat food into Theo's and Cleo's plastic bowls.

Just then the doorbell rang. "Who is it?" Cindy cried, walking towards the door.

"It's me. Open up," a familiar voice said.

Cindy opened the door to find Jamee Wills, another Bluford freshman, staring at her.

"Cindy!" Jamee shouted. "Girl, what're you doing in pajamas? It's time to go to school."

"I'm not going to school," Cindy said firmly. "Why don't you cut too? We can watch TV, and I got popcorn we can stick in the microwave. And there's pizza in the freezer, too. Today on Paula

Poole's show—"

"Cindy! Girl, get it together!" Jamee said, stepping into the apartment. "You need to throw on some clothes and come to school. Keep this up, you gonna be so far behind that you can't do nothin' but fail."

" You don't understand—" Cindy replied, looking down at the worn flip-flops on her feet.

"I understand all right. I understand you gotta get back on track," Jamee replied. "Remember in middle school, Mr. Schuman said you were such a good artist you could be a famous cartoonist for Disney or something? How you gonna be famous if you don't go to school?"

Cindy shrugged. "I can't hang around school all day, Jamee. I get bored. Who cares anyway? My mom wouldn't mind if I quit school. We all just wasting our time in school anyway. Ain't none of us goin' anywhere."

"Cindy, you're crazy," Jamee said, tugging on Cindy's arm. "My sister, Darcy, she's already planning to go to college, and so is her friend Tarah. I'm gonna do the same thing, and you can do it too. But first you gotta get up, change them clothes and get to school. Now come on!"

"Just leave me alone," Cindy insisted.

"Cindy, please come to school."

"Jamee, cut school with me today," Cindy moaned. "If you don't wanna watch TV, I got some CD's we could play and—"

"I'm outta here," Jamee snapped. "I'm not gonna sit here and watch you throw your life away!" Jamee stormed towards the doorway. "When you want to do something with yourself besides sit here watching TV, call me," she said, walking out the door and slamming it behind her. The loud crash of the door was followed by a heavy silence.

Cindy moved to the window and watched Jamee shift her backpack and join the stream of kids heading for Bluford. Part of her wanted to join the crowd and head to school, but another part of her did not want to move. Unlike Jamee and her classmates,

Cindy felt foreign and out of place at school. Her teachers often said she was "quiet" and "shy," but Cindy knew she was just different.

Turning from the window, Cindy grabbed the magazines on the living room floor and stacked them neatly on the coffee table. Then she picked up a pile of dirty clothes she had left sitting on the living room chair for weeks.

"Yuck, these stink!" Cindy groaned. It had been a while since she had washed her laundry. Sometimes she just picked an outfit from the dirty clothes pile to wear to school. As long as things were not too dirty or wrinkled, she would still wear them. It had not always been this way. In fact, Cindy did have a few new clothes that she got for the start of her freshman year. But as weeks passed and her mother spent less and less time at home, laundry, like school, seemed less important.

Glancing around the cluttered living room, Cindy focused on the small picture of her mother that sat next to the TV. Raffie, her mother's boyfriend, was also in the picture, his arm resting on her shoulder like a heavy snake. Only a few months old, the picture captured her mother's flawless milk-chocolate skin and her radiant smile. *Mom is beautiful,* Cindy thought, *and I look nothing like her.* Where her mother was tall, curvy, and attractive, Cindy was long and skinny. But worse than her lanky shape was her nose. To Cindy, it seemed to spread too far across the middle of her face, making her feel that her head was just a platform on which her nose rested.

Friends of her mother had always been kind, but even they noticed how different Cindy was. *"Oh, I can't see a resemblance,"* they would politely begin. *"You must take after your father."* Cindy knew exactly what they were trying to say, but she appreciated their attempt to spare her feelings.

The only person who did not seem concerned with Cindy's feelings was Raffie. *"Are you sure she's your momma?"* he asked Cindy when he began dating her mother last year. When Cindy first met him, he was sitting at the kitchen table, gold chains jangling around his neck, gold earrings glittering from his earlobes, and a smirk on his face.

"You ain't nothin' like your momma," he had said. *"She is what a man would call one hot lady."* Since then, Cindy did her best to ignore Raffie, but it was not easy. Often he said things that made her feel even worse about her looks, but he always did it out of Mom's earshot, calling Cindy "Ugly Mugly" and flaring his nostrils to taunt her. Whenever Cindy asked him to stop, he would laugh in her face. Once, he even flapped his arms in a mock imitation of her long, awkward limbs.

In August, Cindy's mother announced that she and Raffie were "serious," and since then, she spent most of her free time with him. In the rare moments Mom was home, all she could talk about was Raffie. Cindy cringed each time she heard his name. It seemed to her that Raffie was gradually taking over her mother's life. Worse, it appeared as if that was exactly what Mom wanted.

Alone in the apartment, Cindy sat in the recliner in front of the TV and turned it on with the remote control. She had to push hard to make the recliner go back into a comfortable position. The old chair did not work as well as it used to, and Mom said she did not make enough money at her waitressing job to buy a new one.

Cindy had believed her until she noticed her mother frequently buying herself new outfits to wear for Raffie. It seemed that once a week Mom came home carrying shopping bags from expensive department stores. When Cindy asked her about it, Mom explained that Raffie had been giving her money so she could buy nice clothes, but this only made Cindy more upset. It was as if Raffie was buying her mother away from her, and there was nothing Cindy could do to stop it.

Cindy began flipping through the channels when she heard the doorbell ring. Annoyed, she turned toward the door and called out, "Yeah? Who is it?"

"Mrs. Davis, honey," came a familiar voice. Rose Davis lived at the other end of the hall. She was raising her fifteen-year-old grandson, Harold. Once, in the basement laundry room, Cindy overheard Mrs. Davis tell a neighbor that Harold's mother had died in childbirth, and his father never was in the picture.

Cindy got up and opened the door. "Hi, Mrs. Davis."

"Child, I heard the TV goin', so I figured you were home. I was worried about you. Ain't you supposed to be in school?" Mrs. Davis asked.

"Uh . . . I got cramps," Cindy lied, rubbing her hand on her stomach.

"Poor thing! I make tea that's real soothin' for that. I'll bring you some if you like," Mrs. Davis offered.

"No, thank you. I just took something. I'll feel better soon," Cindy said, smiling.

Rose Davis stared at her for a moment. Cindy braced herself for criticism about not being in school. But then the old woman began to smile. "Child, you got the prettiest eyes I ever did see," she said.

"Me?" Cindy said, stunned. "You must be thinkin' of my mom. She's got real pretty eyes with long lashes, but my eyes are—"

"I never noticed before that you got the prettiest hazel-brown eyes, Cindy," Mrs. Davis added. "Folks say the eyes are windows to the soul. They believe you can look someone right in the eye and tell what kind of person they are."

"Some boy in school says I have freak eyes," Cindy said. "Now, him and all his friends call me that whenever they see me."

Mrs. Davis grabbed hold of Cindy's shoulders and looked into her face. "Child, your eyes are beautiful, and don't you forget that. Pay no mind to what a boy says 'bout you. My grandson Harold tells me that some of them kids at your school can be downright nasty sometimes. It's like I tell him—when they start talkin' that nonsense, you just stop listenin.' Let'em call you names. But it's you who's got the prettiest eyes around, not them. Remember that."

As she spoke, Mrs. Davis gently placed her hand on Cindy's cheek. "Some people need to see their own beauty before they can believe they got it," she said, smiling. Mrs. Davis waved goodbye and headed down the long hallway.

Cindy hurried to the bathroom mirror and stared into it. She stood for a long time, moving her face in close for a better look. Her mother had a mirror that magnified everything, and Cindy looked in that too. Her large hazel eyes stared back at her. *Did Mrs. Davis mean what she said, or was she being nice?* Cindy wondered.

Leaving the TV on, Cindy jumped in the shower and washed her hair. Then she gathered her dirty clothes, took them downstairs and put them in the washing machine. When the clothes were dry, she brought them back upstairs, folded them neatly and put them into her drawers. It was the first time she had done her laundry in weeks.

After putting the clothes away, Cindy found a pair of white jeans and two ribbed tank tops, one blue and the other green and yellow. *Maybe I'll go to school tomorrow wearing one of these tank tops,* she thought. Probably not, but if she felt like it in the morning, she might go. Mom would write a note explaining that she had been sick. Mom never seemed to care what excuses Cindy used to skip school. Cindy practically dictated them, always remembering to vary the made-up ailments. She used headaches until a nosy teacher started pushing her to see a doctor. Then she added cramps and fevers to her list of illnesses.

As Cindy thought about returning to school, she again recalled what Mrs. Davis said about her having "the prettiest eyes." She grabbed her mother's magnifying mirror and sat on the recliner looking into it. Cindy tried hard to see what Mrs. Davis saw.

"Maybe my eyes *are* pretty," Cindy said into the mirror.

On Paula Poole's show, two sisters who were married to the same man were screaming at each other. The show kept bleeping out the bad words flying between them, and when they started pulling each other's hair, the audience went wild. Everybody was laughing and cheering.

But Cindy did not pay much attention to the show. She kept staring in the mirror, trying out different expressions to see how they changed the look of her eyes. Maybe she wasn't that bad looking, she thought. With her hair clean and brushed, she didn't think she looked as ugly as Raffie said. And she had clearer skin than most of the other kids at school.

Suddenly the phone rang. Cindy put the mirror down and answered it.

"Hello," she said.

"Yo—who's this?" a familiar deep-throated voice replied. "It's me," Cindy answered. "Oh, Ugly Mugly," Raffie Whitaker said. "How come you home? You get suspended for messin' up at school again?"

"I never been suspended," Cindy corrected him sharply. "And stop calling me that."

Raffie laughed. He always chuckled when he upset Cindy. She could just imagine him on the other end of the line—smiling in satisfaction at how he managed to insult her. "C'mon, Ugly Mugly. Where's your momma?" he asked, still laughing.

"I told you to stop calling me that," Cindy demanded. She wished she could reach into the telephone and wrap the cord around his neck.

"Girl, you so ugly," Raffie went on, in between bursts of cackling laughter, "when the doctor delivered you, he was wearin' a blindfold."

Cindy slammed down the phone. In about a second it rang again. She turned up the TV volume to drown out the ringing. One of the sisters on the Paula Poole show had a nail file, and she looked as if she was about to attack the other one with it. Maybe it was all an act, but the hate in the girl's face seemed real. It was the same hatred Cindy felt for Raffie.

Cindy fantasized about being on the show with Raffie Whitaker. She imagined herself grabbing the gold chains he hung around his neck and pulling them so tight his eyes bulged out.

The phone kept ringing. "I ain't gonna answer you. You can't make me." Cindy smiled because for once she had power. Raffie Whitaker was fuming somewhere , and he could not do a thing about it.

Ignoring the phone's periodic ringing, Cindy picked up the mirror again and repeated the words that Mrs. Davis had said. "Pretty eyes . . . pretty hazel eyes."

Maybe Mrs. Davis was not the only one who thought she was special. Maybe someone else would feel that way about her too one day.

If you'd like to continue reading this book, it is available for $1/copy from TownsendPress.com. Or tell an adult (like your teacher) that they can receive copies of *Someone to Love Me* for free if they order a class set of 15 or more copies of *Am I Ready*. To order, call 212-279-0708 x115 or visit www.youthcomm.org.

Teens:
How to Get More Out of This Book

Self-help: The teens who wrote the stories in this book did so because they hope that telling their stories will help readers who are facing similar challenges. They want you to know that you are not alone, and that taking specific steps can help you manage or overcome very difficult situations. They've done their best to be clear about the actions that worked for them so you can see if they'll work for you.

Writing: You can also use the book to improve your writing skills. Each teen in this book wrote 5-10 drafts of his or her story before it was published. If you read the stories closely you'll see that the teens work to include a beginning, a middle, and an end, and good scenes, description, dialogue, and anecdotes (little stories). To improve your writing, take a look at how these writers construct their stories. Try some of their techniques in your own writing.

Reading: Finally, you'll notice that we include the first chapter from a Bluford Series novel in this book, alongside the true stories by teens. We hope you'll like it enough to continue reading. The more you read, the more you'll strengthen your reading skills. Teens at Youth Communication like the Bluford novels because they explore themes similar to those in their own stories. Your school may already have the Bluford books. If not, you can order them online for only $1.

Resources on the Web

We will occasionally post Think About It questions on our website, www.youthcomm.org, to accompany stories in this and other Youth Communication books. We try out the questions with teens and post the ones they like best. Many teens report that writing answers to those questions in a journal is very helpful.

How to Use This Book in Staff Training

Staff say that reading these stories gives them greater insight into what teens are thinking and feeling, and new strategies for working with them. You can help the staff you work with by using these stories as case studies.

Select one story to read in the group, and ask staff to identify and discuss the main issue facing the teen. There may be disagreement about this, based on the background and experience of staff. That is fine. One point of the exercise is that teens have complex lives and needs. Adults can probably be more effective if they don't focus too narrowly and can see several dimensions of their clients.

Ask staff: What issues or feelings does the story provoke in them? What kind of help do they think the teen wants? What interventions are likely to be most promising? Least effective? Why? How would you build trust with the teen writer? How have other adults failed the teen, and how might that affect his or her willingness to accept help? What other resources would be helpful to this teen, such as peer support, a mentor, counseling, family therapy, etc?

Resources on the Web

From time to time we will post Think About It questions on our website, www.youthcomm.org, to accompany stories in this and other Youth Communication books. We try out the questions with teens and post the ones that they find most effective. We'll also post lessons for some of the stories. Adults can use the questions and lessons in workshops.

| Discussion Guide |

Teachers and Staff:
How to Use This Book in Groups

When working with teens individually or in groups, you can use these stories to help young people face difficult issues in a way that feels safe to them. That's because talking about the issues in the stories usually feels safer to teens than talking about those same issues in their own lives. Addressing issues through the stories allows for some personal distance; they hit close to home, but not too close. Talking about them opens up a safe place for reflection. As teens gain confidence talking about the issues in the stories, they usually become more comfortable talking about those issues in their own lives.

Below are general questions to guide your discussion. In most cases you can read a story and conduct a discussion in one 45-minute session. Teens are usually happy to read the stories aloud, with each teen reading a paragraph or two. (Allow teens to pass if they don't want to read.) It takes 10-15 minutes to read a story straight through. However, it is often more effective to let workshop participants make comments and discuss the story as you go along. The workshop leader may even want to annotate her copy of the story beforehand with key questions.

If teens read the story ahead of time or silently, it's good to break the ice with a few questions that get everyone on the same page: Who is the main character? How old is she? What happened to her? How did she respond? Another good starting question is: "What stood out for you in the story?" Go around the room and let each person briefly mention one thing.

Then move on to open-ended questions, which encourage participants to think more deeply about what the writers were feeling, the choices they faced, and the actions they took. There are no right or wrong answers to the open-ended questions.

Open-ended questions encourage participants to think about how the themes, emotions, and choices in the stories relate to their own lives. Here are some examples of open-ended questions that we have found to be effective. You can use variations of these questions with almost any story in this book.

—What main problem or challenge did the writer face?

—What choices did the teen have in trying to deal with the problem?

—Which way of dealing with the problem was most effective for the teen? Why?

—What strengths, skills, or resources did the teen use to address the challenge?

—If you were in the writer's shoes, what would you have done?

—What could adults have done better to help this young person?

—What have you learned by reading this story that you didn't know before?

—What, if anything, will you do differently after reading this story?

—What surprised you in this story?

—Do you have a different view of this issue, or see a different way of dealing with it, after reading this story? Why or why not?

Credits

The stories in this book originally appeared in the following Youth Communication publications:

"Womanhood Can Wait," by Nicole Hawkins, *New Youth Connections*, September/October 1998; "I Stopped Giving in to Him," by Anonymous, *New Youth Connections*, September/October 1996; "When It Comes to Dating, Older Isn't Better," by Shaniece McKenzie, *New Youth Connections*, May/June 1998; "Communication Is More Important Than Sex," by Anonymous, *New Youth Connections*, March 2007; "Virgin Under Pressure," by Anonymous, *New Youth Connections*, December 2003; "The Morning After," by Anonymous, *New Youth Connections*, May/June 2002; "Looking for Love," by Fetima P., *Represent*, May/June 1998; "I Need a Girl," by Destiny, *New Youth Connections*, May/June 2002; "All Men Are Dawgs," by Wunika Hicks, *Represent*, January/February 1995; "I Was Scared but I Wanted Experience," by Anonymous, *New Youth Connections*, March 2003; "Can We Talk About Sex With Our Parents?" by Anonymous, *New Youth Connections*, March 2006; "Dirty Dancing," by Janill Briones, *New Youth Connections*, April 2005; "It Takes Love to Make Love," by Anonymous, *New Youth Connections*, November 2005; "Single, Happy, and Free," by Irma Johnson, *New Youth Connections*, September/October 1991; "The Right Choice—for Now," by Anonymous, *New Youth Connections*, September/October 1999; "Scare Tactics," by Anonymous, *New Youth Connections*, January/February 2000; "I Paid the Price for Unprotected Sex—Twice," by Anonymous, *New Youth Connections*, March 1999.

About
Youth Communication

Youth Communication, founded in 1980, is a nonprofit youth development program located in New York City whose mission is to teach writing, journalism, and leadership skills. The teenagers we train become writers for our websites and books and for two print magazines: *New Youth Connections*, a general-interest youth magazine, and *Represent*, a magazine by and for young people in foster care.

Each year, up to 100 young people participate in Youth Communication's school-year and summer journalism workshops, where they work under the direction of full-time professional editors. Most are African-American, Latino, or Asian, and many are recent immigrants. The opportunity to reach their peers with accurate portrayals of their lives and important self-help information motivates the young writers to create powerful stories.

Our goal is to run a strong youth development program in which teens produce high quality stories that inform and inspire their peers. Doing so requires us to be sensitive to the complicated lives and emotions of the teen participants while also providing an intellectually rigorous experience. We achieve that goal in the writing/teaching/editing relationship, which is the core of our program.

Our teaching and editorial process begins with discussions

between adult editors and the teen staff. In those meetings, the teens and the editors work together to identify the most important issues in the teens' lives and to figure out how those issues can be turned into stories that will resonate with teen readers.

Once story topics are chosen, students begin the process of crafting their stories. For a personal story, that means revisiting events in one's past to understand their significance for the future. For a commentary, it means developing a logical and persuasive point of view. For a reported story, it means gathering information through research and interviews. Students look inward and outward as they try to make sense of their experiences and the world around them and find the points of intersection between personal and social concerns. That process can take a few weeks or a few months. Stories frequently go through ten or more drafts as students work under the guidance of their editors, the way any professional writer does.

Many of the students who walk through our doors have uneven skills, as a result of poor education, living under extremely stressful conditions, or coming from homes where English is a second language. Yet, to complete their stories, students must successfully perform a wide range of activities, including writing and rewriting, reading, discussion, reflection, research, interviewing, and typing. They must work as members of a team and they must accept individual responsibility. They learn to provide constructive criticism, and to accept it. They engage in explorations of truthfulness, fairness, and accuracy. They meet deadlines. They must develop the audacity to believe that they have something important to say and the humility to recognize that saying it well is not a process of instant gratification. Rather, it usually requires a long, hard struggle through many discussions and much rewriting.

It would be impossible to teach these skills and dispositions as separate, disconnected topics, like grammar, ethics, or assertiveness. However, we find that students make rapid progress when they are learning skills in the context of an inquiry that is personally significant to them and that will benefit their peers.

When teens publish their stories—in *New Youth Connections* and *Represent*, on the Web, and in other publications—they reach tens of thousands of teen and adult readers. Teachers, counselors, social workers, and other adults circulate the stories to young people in their classes and out-of-school youth programs. Adults tell us that teens in their programs—including many who are ordinarily resistant to reading—clamor for the stories. Teen readers report that the stories give them information they can't get anywhere else, and inspire them to reflect on their lives and open lines of communication with adults.

Writers usually participate in our program for one semester, though some stay much longer. Years later, many of them report that working here was a turning point in their lives—that it helped them acquire the confidence and skills that they needed for success in college and careers. Scores of our graduates have overcome tremendous obstacles to become journalists, writers, and novelists. They include National Book Award finalist and MacArthur Fellowship winner Edwidge Danticat, novelist Ernesto Quiñonez, writer Veronica Chambers, and *New York Times* reporter Rachel Swarns. Hundreds more are working in law, business, and other careers. Many are teachers, principals, and youth workers, and several have started nonprofit youth programs themselves and work as mentors—helping another generation of young people develop their skills and find their voices.

Youth Communication is a nonprofit educational corporation. Contributions are gratefully accepted and are tax deductible to the fullest extent of the law.

To make a contribution, or for information about our publications and programs, including our catalog of over 100 books and curricula for hard-to-reach teens, see www.youthcomm.org.

About the Editors

Virginia Vitzthum is an editor at *Represent*, Youth Communication's magazine by and for teens in foster care. Before working at Youth Communication she wrote a book about Internet dating and a column for the Web magazine salon.com. She's also written for *Ms.*, *Elle, the Village Voice, Time Out New York, Washington City Paper*, and other publications. She has edited law books, books about substance abuse treatment, and health care policy newsletters. She's written a play and a screenplay; produced several short videos; and volunteered at the 52nd St. Project, a children's theater, where she helped 9- to 11-year-olds write plays.

Keith Hefner co-founded Youth Communication in 1980 and has directed it ever since. He is the recipient of the Luther P. Jackson Education Award from the New York Association of Black Journalists and a MacArthur Fellowship. He was also a Revson Fellow at Columbia University.

Laura Longhine is the editorial director at Youth Communication. She edited *Represent*, Youth Communication's magazine by and for youth in foster care, for three years, and has written for a variety of publications. She has a BA in English from Tufts University and an MS in Journalism from Columbia University.

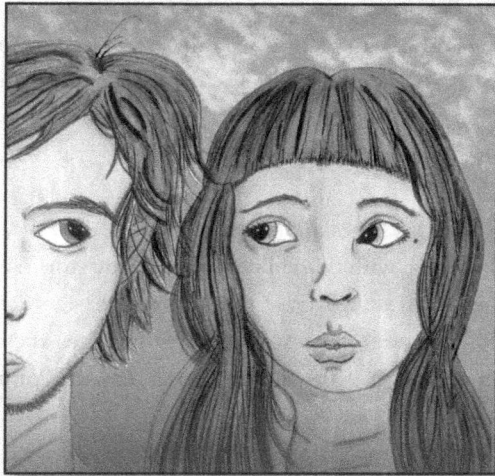

More Helpful Books
From Youth Communication

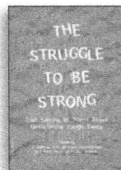

The Struggle to Be Strong: True Stories by Teens About Overcoming Tough Times. Foreword by Veronica Chambers. Help young people identify and build on their own strengths with 30 personal stories about resiliency. (Free Spirit)

Starting With "I": Personal Stories by Teenagers. "Who am I and who do I want to become?" Thirty-five stories examine this question through the lens of race, ethnicity, gender, sexuality, family, and more. Increase this book's value with the free Teacher's Guide, available from youthcomm.org. (Youth Communication)

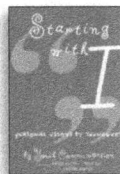

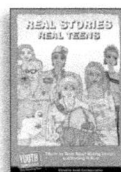

Real Stories, Real Teens. Inspire teens to read and recognize their strengths with this collection of 26 true stories by teens. The young writers describe how they overcame significant challenges and stayed true to themselves. Also includes the first chapters from three novels in the Bluford Series. (Youth Communication)

The Courage to Be Yourself: True Stories by Teens About Cliques, Conflicts, and Overcoming Peer Pressure. In 26 first-person stories, teens write about their lives with searing honesty. These stories will inspire young readers to reflect on their own lives, work through their problems, and help them discover who they really are. (Free Spirit)

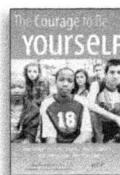

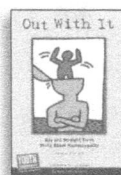

Out With It: Gay and Straight Teens Write About Homosexuality. Break stereotypes and provide support with this unflinching look at gay life from a teen's perspective. With a focus on urban youth, this book also includes several heterosexual teens' transformative experiences with gay peers. (Youth Communication)

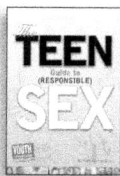

The Teen Guide to (Responsible) Sex. Help teens understand that sex isn't something that just happens to them—they have choices. This book offers thoughtful questions teens should ask themselves if they're considering having sex—plus honest accounts from peers who describe how becoming sexually active has changed their lives, for better or worse. (Youth Communication)

From Dropout to Achiever: Teens Write About School. Help teens overcome the challenges of graduating, which may involve overcoming family problems, bouncing back from a bad semester, or even dropping out for a time. These teens show how they achieve academic success. (Youth Communication)

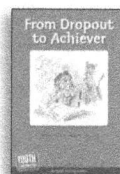

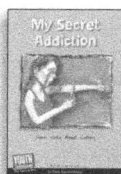

My Secret Addiction: Teens Write About Cutting. These true accounts of cutting, or self-mutilation, offer a window into the personal and family situations that lead to this secret habit, and show how teens can get the help they need. (Youth Communication)

Why I'm Still a Virgin: Teens Write About Saying No to Sex (Or Wishing They Had). Teens share why they have chosen to abstain from sex, often in the face of extreme peer pressure. They have a variety of reasons—fear, religion, morals, family values, or just a personal sense that they're not ready. (Youth Communication)

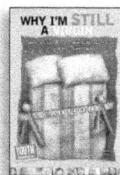

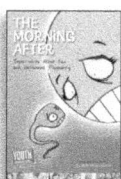

The Morning After: Teens Write About Sex and Unplanned Pregnancy. Help prevent unplanned pregnancy with these true stories by teens who have been there. A comprehensive guide to birth control is also included. (Youth Communication)

Through Thick and Thin: Teens Write About Obesity, Eating Disorders, and Self Image. Help teens who struggle with obesity, eating disorders, and body weight issues. These stories show the pressures teens face when they are confronted by unrealistic standards for physical appearance, and how emotions can affect the way we eat. (Youth Communication)

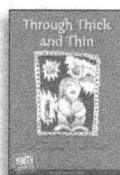

To order these and other books, go to:
www.youthcomm.org
or call 212-279-0708 x115

www.ingramcontent.com/pod-product-compliance
Lightning Source LLC
Chambersburg PA
CBHW052219270326
41931CB00011B/2416